DIABETES INSTANT POT COOKBOOK FOR BEGINNERS

Nourishing Simplicity: Enjoy 200+ Diabetic-Friendly Easy Home Cooked Recipes to Manage Blood Sugar

KELLY WALTERHOUSE

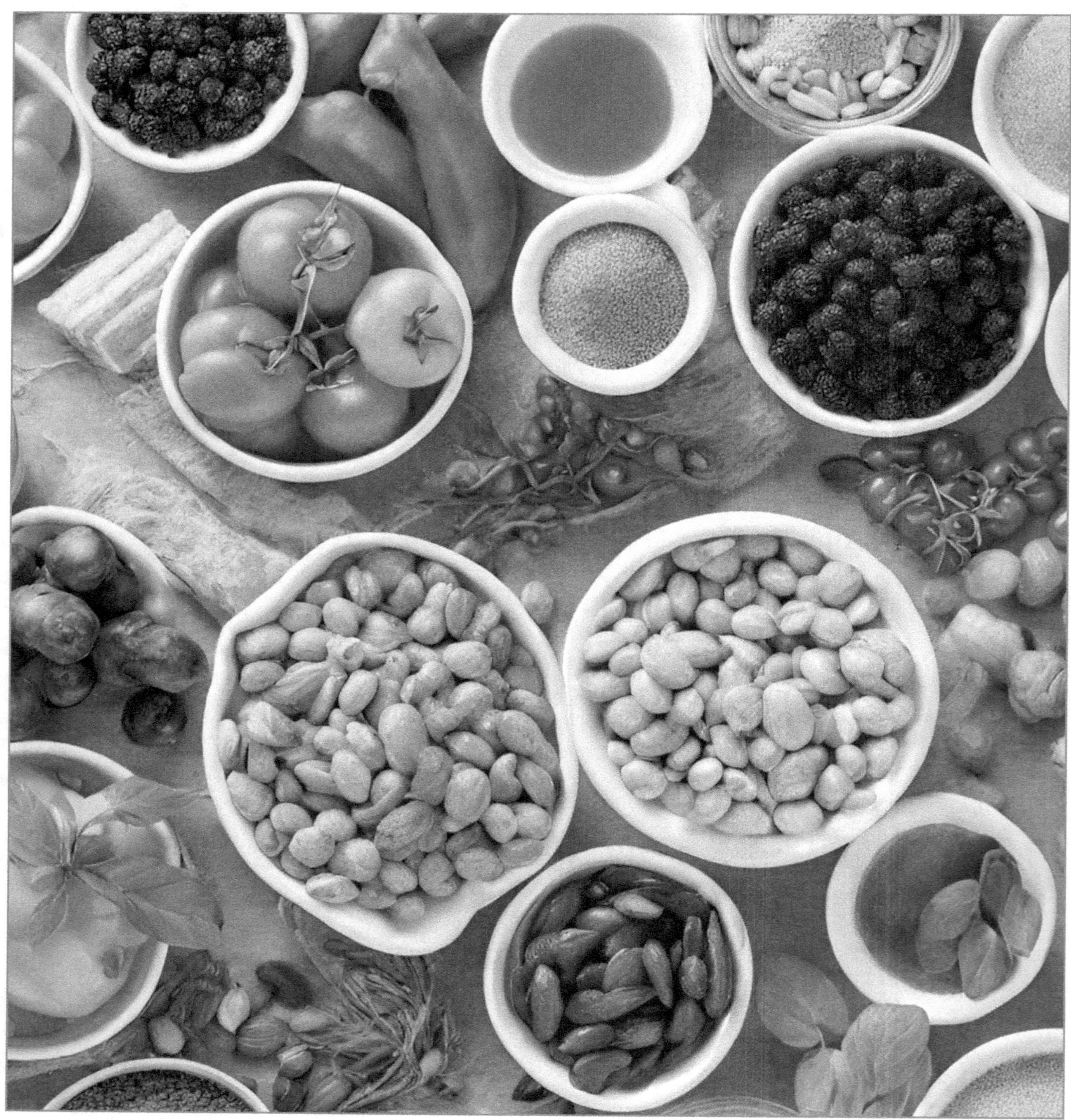

2 Diabetes Instant Pot Cookbook For Beginners

Table of Content

5 Diabetes Instant Pot Cookbook For Beginners

6 Diabetes Instant Pot Cookbook For Beginners

8 Diabetes Instant Pot Cookbook For Beginners

9 Diabetes Instant Pot Cookbook For Beginners

Introduction

In the fast paced world of modern cooking, the Instant Pot has emerged as a revolutionary kitchen appliance, transforming the way people approach meal preparation. This multifunctional electric pressure cooker has gained immense popularity for its efficiency, timesaving capabilities, and versatility in preparing a wide range of dishes. As we delve into the realm of diabetic friendly recipes tailored for the Instant Pot, it's essential to first understand the significance of this culinary marvel.

Brief Overview of the Instant Pot

The Instant Pot, often referred to as the "kitchen magician," combines several kitchen appliances into one, functioning as a pressure cooker, slow cooker, rice cooker, steamer, sauté pan, and even a yogurt maker. Its ability to perform multiple cooking tasks with precision and speed has turned it into a beloved asset for both novice and seasoned cooks. The appliance's sealed cooking environment not only reduces cooking times but also preserves the nutritional value of ingredients, making it an ideal companion for health conscious individuals.

The Instant Pot operates by creating a high-pressure environment that raises the boiling point of liquids, resulting in faster cooking times. This method is particularly advantageous for individuals with diabetes who need to carefully manage their diet, as it allows for the preparation of nutritious meals in a shorter duration, minimizing the impact on blood sugar levels.

Importance of Diabetic Friendly Recipes

As diabetes continues to be a prevalent health concern globally, there is a growing need for culinary solutions that cater to individuals managing this condition. The importance of diabetic friendly recipes cannot be overstated, as they play a pivotal role in promoting balanced nutrition, maintaining stable blood sugar levels, and enhancing overall wellbeing.

One of the primary challenges for people with diabetes is navigating a landscape of dietary restrictions while still enjoying flavorful and satisfying meals. Traditional cooking methods may not always align with the dietary requirements of individuals managing diabetes, leading to a quest for innovative and efficient cooking solutions. This is where the Instant Pot steps in, offering a platform to create delicious and diabetes friendly dishes without compromising on taste or nutritional value.

Diabetic friendly recipes crafted for the Instant Pot focus on incorporating ingredients with lower glycemic indexes, reducing added sugars, and increasing fiber content. The controlled cooking environment of the Instant Pot ensures that flavors are intensified, allowing for the use of fewer seasonings and healthier cooking techniques. This approach not only caters to the dietary needs of those with diabetes but also contributes to promoting a healthy lifestyle for everyone.

Moreover, the convenience of the Instant Pot aligns with the busy lifestyles that many individuals lead today. The time efficient nature of pressure cooking makes it easier for people to adhere to their dietary plans without sacrificing culinary enjoyment. This is especially crucial for those managing diabetes, where consistency in meal planning and preparation is key to maintaining stable blood sugar levels.

The Instant Pot's ability to infuse flavors into dishes quickly also opens up a world of possibilities for incorporating a variety of nutrient dense foods. From vibrant vegetables to lean proteins, the Instant Pot allows for the creation of diverse and satisfying meals that cater to the specific nutritional requirements of individuals with diabetes.

In summary, the intersection of the Instant Pot and diabetic friendly recipes signifies a harmonious blend of culinary innovation and health conscious cooking. This cookbook aims to explore this intersection, providing a comprehensive guide to creating meals that not only meet the dietary needs of individuals with diabetes but also celebrate the joy of flavorful and nourishing cuisine.

Instant Pot Basics

The Instant Pot, often hailed as a kitchen game changer, has become an indispensable tool for many households seeking efficiency and versatility in their culinary endeavors. To fully harness the potential of this multifunctional appliance, a fundamental understanding of Instant Pot basics is essential. In this section, we will delve into a comprehensive guide on using the Instant Pot and explore valuable tips for adapting recipes to cater specifically to the dietary needs of individuals managing diabetes.

Guide to Using the Instant Pot

1. Getting Acquainted with the Instant Pot:

The Instant Pot typically comes with several preset cooking functions, including pressure cooking, slow cooking, sautéing, and more. Familiarize yourself with the control panel, buttons, and the corresponding functions. Understanding the nuances of each setting will enable you to leverage the Instant Pot's versatility.

2. Assembling and Disassembling:

Start by assembling the Instant Pot correctly, ensuring that the sealing ring is in place and the inner pot is securely positioned. Familiarize yourself with the steam release valve, float valve, and other components. Proper disassembly is crucial for thorough cleaning and maintenance.

3. Pressure Cooking Basics:

The hallmark feature of the Instant Pot is its pressure cooking capability. Master the art of using high and low pressure settings based on your recipe requirements. The Instant Pot's sealed cooking environment allows for faster cooking times while preserving the flavors and nutrients of the ingredients.

4. Sautéing and Browning:

The sauté function adds a versatile dimension to your cooking. Use it to brown meats, sauté vegetables, or develop flavors before pressure cooking. This step enhances the depth of taste in your dishes, contributing to a well-rounded culinary experience.

5. Understanding Release Methods:

After pressure cooking, familiarize yourself with the natural release and quick release methods. Natural release allows pressure to subside gradually, ideal for delicate dishes, while quick release rapidly releases pressure, suitable for recipes where overcooking is a concern.

6. Utilizing Accessories:

The Instant Pot supports various accessories such as steam racks, trivets, and silicone molds. These accessories enhance cooking versatility, enabling you to prepare multiple components simultaneously or cook dishes like cheesecakes and egg bites with ease.

7. Cleaning and Maintenance:

Regular cleaning is crucial for the longevity of your Instant Pot. The removable parts, including the sealing ring and steam release valve, should be cleaned thoroughly after each use. Refer to the manufacturer's guidelines for maintenance and troubleshooting.

8. Experimenting and Adapting:

The Instant Pot encourages experimentation. Don't hesitate to adapt traditional recipes for this appliance. Whether it's converting slow cooker recipes or exploring new cuisines, the Instant Pot's adaptability opens doors to a world of culinary possibilities.

Understanding Diabetes and Nutrition

In the intricate tapestry of health management, a crucial thread is dedicated to understanding diabetes and its intricate relationship with nutrition. As we embark on a journey into the basics of diabetes management and nutritional considerations for individuals grappling with this condition, it becomes evident that the synergy between what we eat and how our bodies respond is paramount.

Basics of Diabetes Management

Diabetes, a chronic condition characterized by elevated blood sugar levels, demands a vigilant and proactive approach to management. The body's inability to produce enough insulin or effectively use the insulin it produces lies at the core of diabetes. Insulin, a hormone produced by the pancreas, regulates blood sugar by facilitating the absorption of glucose into cells. When this delicate balance is disrupted, it necessitates a comprehensive management strategy.

Understanding diabetes involves recognizing the different types – Type 1, where the body doesn't produce insulin, and Type 2, where the body doesn't use insulin properly. Both types require attention to diet, physical activity, medication (if prescribed), and regular monitoring of blood sugar levels. The objective is to maintain blood sugar within a target range, preventing complications that can affect the heart, kidneys, eyes, and nerves.

One of the cornerstones of diabetes management is adopting a mindful and balanced approach to nutrition. This is where the significance of choosing the right foods and understanding their impact on blood sugar levels comes into play.

Understanding the nuances of diabetes management and nutritional considerations empowers individuals to make informed choices that positively impact their health. The Instant Pot, with its ability to facilitate the preparation of wholesome and balanced meals, becomes an invaluable tool in this journey toward optimal wellbeing.

Tips for Adapting Recipes for Diabetes

Let's delve into valuable tips for adapting recipes to meet the specific dietary requirements of individuals with diabetes:

1. Mindful Carbohydrate Choices:

Opt for whole grains, legumes, and vegetables with a low glycemic index in your Instant Pot recipes. This ensures a slower release of glucose into the bloodstream, promoting better blood sugar control.

2. Sugar Substitutes:

Explore natural sugar substitutes like stevia, erythritol, or monk fruit in place of refined sugars. This allows you to enjoy a touch of sweetness in your Instant Pot desserts without compromising on diabetic friendly principles.

3. Lean Proteins:

Choose lean protein sources such as poultry, fish, tofu, or legumes for your Instant Pot recipes. These proteins contribute to satiety without the excess saturated fats often associated with certain cuts of meat.

4. Balancing Macronutrients:

Ensure a well-balanced distribution of macronutrients in your Instant Pot meals. Combining proteins, healthy fats, and complex carbohydrates promotes sustained energy levels and helps manage blood sugar fluctuations.

5. Portion Control:

Leverage the Instant Pot's precision in portioning to create well-balanced meals. Controlling portion sizes is a key aspect of diabetes management, and the Instant Pot facilitates this by allowing for accurate measurements.

6. Herbs and Spices for Flavor:

Enhance the flavor profile of your Instant Pot dishes with herbs and spices rather than relying on excessive salt or sugar. This not only adds depth to your recipes but also aligns with a heart healthy and diabetes friendly approach to cooking.

7. Monitoring Sodium Intake:

Be mindful of sodium content in your Instant Pot recipes. Opt for low sodium broth or sauces and use herbs and spices creatively to season your dishes. Managing sodium intake is essential for overall health, especially for individuals with diabetes.

8. Experimenting with Whole Food Ingredients:

Incorporate whole foods into your Instant Pot recipes. Fresh vegetables, lean proteins, and unprocessed ingredients contribute to a nutrient dense and diabetes friendly approach to cooking.

9. Using Low-fat Dairy:

When a recipe calls for dairy, opt for low-fat or fat free varieties. This reduces the overall saturated fat content of your Instant Pot dishes while still providing the creamy texture associated with certain recipes.

16 Diabetes Instant Pot Cookbook For Beginners

10. Monitoring Cooking Times:

The Instant Pot's efficiency in reducing cooking times is advantageous, but it also requires careful monitoring. Avoid overcooking ingredients, especially those with higher sugar content, to preserve their texture and prevent unnecessary caramelization.

By combining the versatility of the Instant Pot with these diabetes conscious tips, you can create a diverse array of flavorful, satisfying, and health conscious meals. The marriage of convenience and nutritional mindfulness embodied by the Instant Pot makes it a valuable ally in the pursuit of delicious, diabetes friendly cooking.

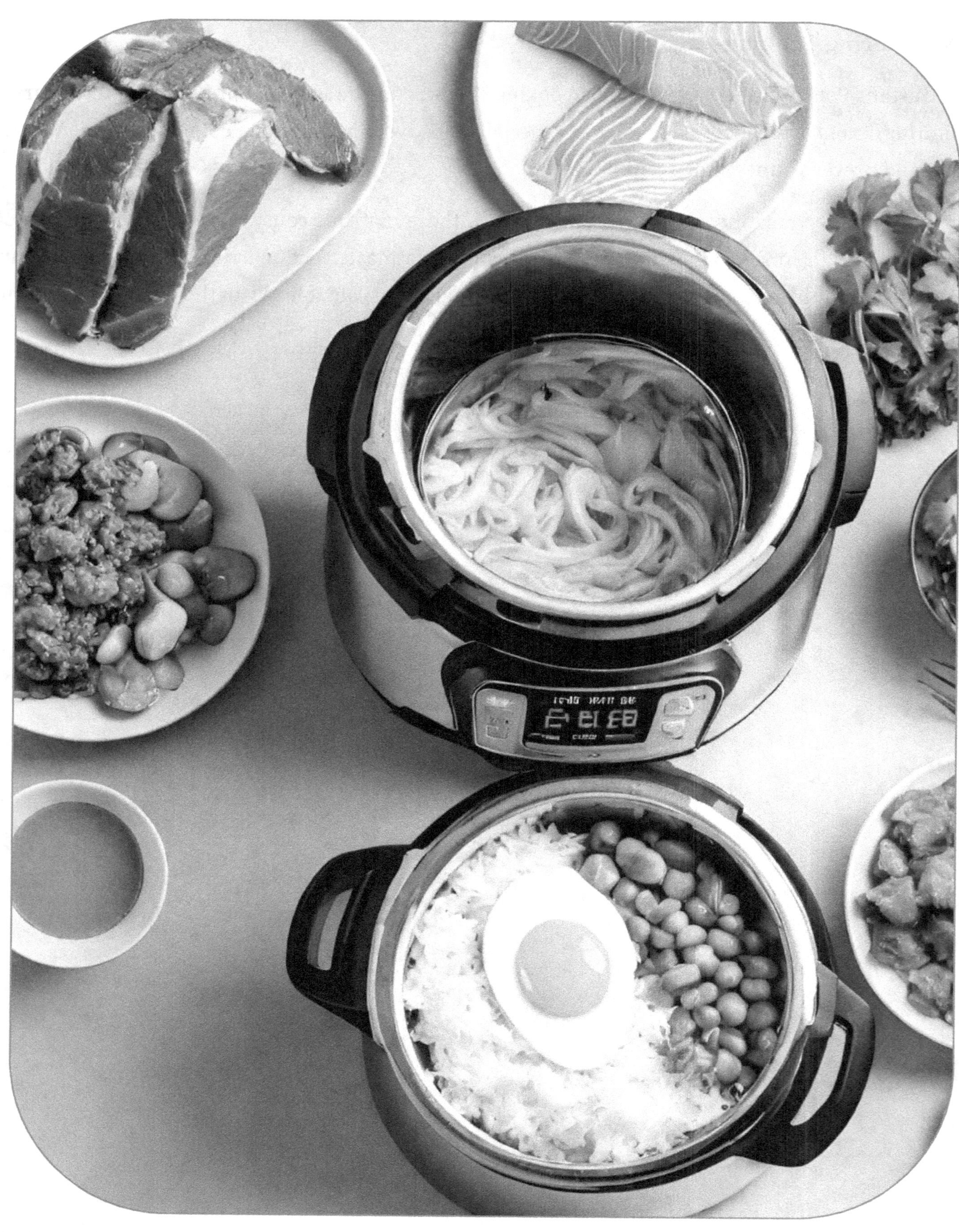

18 Diabetes Instant Pot Cookbook For Beginners

BREAKFAST

STEEL CUT OATS

Prep Time: 5 minutes Servings: 4

Nutrition per Serving: 150 calories, 3g protein, 30g carbohydrates, 2g fat, 5g fiber

Ingredients:

- 1 cup steel cut oats
- 3 cups water
- 1/2 teaspoon cinnamon
- Fresh berries for topping

Instructions:

1. Combine oats, water, and cinnamon in the Instant Pot.
2. Cook on high pressure for 10 minutes, then allow a natural release.
3. Serve with fresh berries.

VEGETABLE FRITTATA

Prep Time: 15 minutes Servings: 6

Nutrition per Serving: 120 Calories, 10g protein, 5g carbohydrates, 7g fat, 2g fiber

Ingredients:

- 6 eggs, beaten
- 1 cup diced bell peppers
- 1 cup diced zucchini
- 1/2 cup diced onion
- Salt and pepper to taste

Instructions:

1. Sauté vegetables in the Instant Pot.
2. Pour beaten eggs over the vegetables.
3. Cook on high pressure for 5 minutes. Quick release and serve.

GREEK YOGURT PARFAIT

Prep Time: 10 minutes Servings: 2

Nutrition per Serving: 200 calories, 15g protein, 20g carbohydrates, 8g fat, 2g fiber

Ingredients:

- 2 cups plain Greek yogurt
- 1 cup mixed berries
- 1 tablespoon honey
- 2 tablespoons chopped nuts

Instructions:

1. Layer Greek yogurt, berries, honey, and nuts in a bowl or jar.
2. Repeat layers.
3. Enjoy chilled.

QUINOA BREAKFAST BOWL

Prep Time: 10 minutes Servings: 4

Nutrition per Serving: 180 calories, 6g protein, 30g carbohydrates, 4g fat, 3g fiber

Ingredients:

- 1 cup quinoa, rinsed
- 2 cups water
- 1 cup almond milk
- 1 teaspoon vanilla extract
- Fresh fruit for topping

Instructions:

2. Combine quinoa, water, almond milk, and vanilla in the Instant Pot.
3. Cook on high pressure for 1 minute.

1. Allow a natural release. Top with fresh fruit.

LEMON POPPY SEED INSTANT POT MUFFINS

Prep Time: 15 minutes Servings: 8

Nutrition per Serving: 160 calories, 4g protein, 20g carbohydrates, 8g fat, 2g fiber

Ingredients:

- 1 cup almond flour
- 1/4 cup coconut flour
- 1/4 cup poppy seeds
- 1 teaspoon baking powder
- Zest of 1 lemon

Instructions:

1. Mix ingredients in a bowl.
2. Pour batter into silicone muffin cups.
3. Place cups on a trivet in the Instant Pot.
4. Cook on high pressure for 15 minutes. Quick release.

EGG MUFFINS

Prep Time: 10 minutes   Servings: 4

Nutrition per Serving: 120 calories, 12g protein, 2g carbohydrates, 8g fat, 1g fiber

Ingredients:

- 6 eggs, beaten
- 1 cup chopped spinach
- 1/2 cup diced tomatoes
- 1/4 cup grated Parmesan cheese

Instructions:

1. Mix ingredients in a bowl.
2. Pour into silicone muffin cups.
3. Place cups on a trivet in the Instant Pot.
4. Cook on high pressure for 8 minutes. Quick release.

CINNAMON APPLE QUINOA BOWL

Prep Time: 15 minutes Servings: 4

Nutrition per Serving: 220 calories, 5g protein, 40g carbohydrates, 4g fat, 5g fiber

Ingredients:

- 1 cup quinoa, rinsed
- 2 cups water
- 1 teaspoon cinnamon
- 1 apple, diced
- 2 tablespoons chopped walnuts

Instructions:

1. Combine quinoa, water, and cinnamon in the Instant Pot.
2. Cook on high pressure for 1 minute.
3. Allow a natural release.
4. Top with diced apples and walnuts.

BERRY OATMEAL

Prep Time: 10 minutes Servings: 4

Nutrition per Serving: 180 calories, 6g protein, 30g carbohydrates, 4g fat, 5g fiber

Ingredients:

- 1 cup rolled oats
- 2 cups water
- 1 cup mixed berries (fresh or frozen)
- 1 tablespoon chia seeds

Instructions:

1. Combine oats, water, berries, and chia seeds in the Instant Pot.
2. Cook on high pressure for 3 minutes. Quick release

CHIA SEED PUDDING

Prep Time: 5 minutes (plus chilling time) Servings: 4

Nutrition per Serving: 120 calories, 4g protein, 10g carbohydrates, 8g fat, 6g fiber

Ingredients:

- 1/2 cup chia seeds
- 2 cups unsweetened almond milk
- 1 teaspoon vanilla extract
- Berries for topping

Instructions:

1. Mix chia seeds, almond milk, and vanilla in the Instant Pot.
2. Refrigerate for at least 2 hours or overnight. Top with berries before serving.

COTTAGE CHEESE PANCAKES

Prep Time: 15 minutes Servings: 4

Nutrition per Serving: 160 calories, 12g protein, 15g carbohydrates, 6g fat, 2g fiber

Ingredients:

- 1 cup lowfat cottage cheese
- 4 eggs
- 1/2 cup oat flour
- 1 teaspoon baking powder

Instructions:

1. Blend cottage cheese, eggs, oat flour, and baking powder until smooth
2. . Cook on a greased Instant Pot trivet for 10 minutes on high pressure.

BANANA WALNUT BREAD OATMEAL

Prep Time: 10 minutes Servings: 4

Nutrition per Serving: 220 calories, 6g protein, 35g carbohydrates, 6g fat, 5g fiber

Ingredients:

- 1 cup steelcut oats
- 2 ripe bananas, mashed
- 1/2 cup chopped walnuts
- 1 teaspoon cinnamon

Instructions:

1. Combine oats, mashed bananas, walnuts, and cinnamon in the Instant Pot
2. . Cook on high pressure for 8 minutes.
3. Quick release.

EGG AND SPINACH BREAKFAST CASSEROLE

Prep Time: 15 minutes   Servings: 6

Nutrition per Serving: 150 calories, 14g protein, 5g carbohydrates, 8g fat, 2g fiber

Ingredients:

- 8 eggs, beaten
- 2 cups fresh spinach, chopped
- 1 cup cherry tomatoes, halved
- 1/2 cup feta cheese, crumbled

Instructions:

1. Mix eggs, spinach, tomatoes, and feta in the Instant Pot.
2. Cook on high pressure for 7 minutes. Quick release.

PUMPKIN SPICE OATMEAL

Prep Time: 10 minutes Servings: 4

Nutrition per Serving: 180 calories, 5g protein, 30g carbohydrates, 4g fat, 5g fiber

Ingredients:

- 1 cup rolled oats
- 2 cups water
- 1/2 cup canned pumpkin puree
- 1 teaspoon pumpkin spice

Instructions:

1. Combine oats, water, pumpkin puree, and pumpkin spice in the Instant Pot.
2. Cook on high pressure for 3 minutes. Quick release.

SWEET POTATO BREAKFAST HASH

Prep Time: 15 minutes Servings: 4

Nutrition per Serving: 200 calories, 8g protein, 30g carbohydrates, 6g fat, 5g fiber

Ingredients:

- 2 sweet potatoes, diced
- 1 cup black beans, cooked
- 1 bell pepper, diced
- 1 teaspoon cumin

Instructions:

1. Sauté sweet potatoes, black beans, bell pepper, and cumin in the Instant Pot.
2. Cook on high pressure for 5 minutes. Quick release.

BLUEBERRY ALMOND BREAKFAST QUINOA

Prep Time: 10 minutes   Servings: 4

Nutrition per Serving: 190 calories, 8g protein, 30g carbohydrates, 5g fat, 4g fiber

Ingredients:

- 1 cup quinoa, rinsed
- 2 cups water
- 1 cup blueberries
- 2 tablespoons sliced almonds

Instructions:

1. Combine quinoa, water, blueberries, and almonds in the Instant Pot.
2. Cook on high pressure for 1 minute.
3. Allow a natural release.

SPINACH AND MUSHROOM FRITTATA

Prep Time: 15 minutes   Servings: 6

Nutrition per Serving: 130 calories, 10g protein, 5g carbohydrates, 8g fat, 2g fiber

Ingredients:

- 8 eggs, beaten
- 2 cups fresh spinach, chopped
- 1 cup mushrooms, sliced
- 1/2 cup feta cheese, crumbled

Instructions:

1. Sauté spinach and mushrooms in the Instant Pot.
2. Pour beaten eggs over the vegetables.
3. Cook on high pressure for 7 minutes. Quick release.

CINNAMON RAISIN QUINOA

Prep Time: 10 minutes Servings: 4

Nutrition per Serving: 180 calories, 6g protein, 30g carbohydrates, 4g fat, 3g fiber

Ingredients:

- 1 cup quinoa, rinsed
- 2 cups water
- 1/2 cup raisins
- 1 teaspoon cinnamon

Instructions:

1. Combine quinoa, water, raisins, and cinnamon in the Instant Pot
2. . Cook on high pressure for 1 minute. Allow a natural release.

AVOCADO AND TOMATO EGG CUPS

Prep Time: 10 minutes Servings: 4

Nutrition per Serving: 140 calories, 7g protein, 5g carbohydrates, 10g fat, 3g fiber

Ingredients:

- 4 eggs
- 1 avocado, sliced
- 1 cup cherry tomatoes, halved
- Fresh cilantro for garnish

Instructions:

1. Place avocado slices and cherry tomatoes in Instant Pot silicone molds.
2. Crack an egg into each mold.
3. Cook on high pressure for 5 minutes. Quick release.

APPLE CINNAMON BREAKFAST RICE PUDDING

Prep Time: 15 minutes Servings: 4

Nutrition per Serving: 220 calories, 5g protein, 40g carbohydrates, 5g fat, 3g fiber

Ingredients:

- 1 cup Arborio rice
- 2 cups unsweetened almond milk
- 1 apple, diced
- 1 teaspoon cinnamon

Instructions:

1. Combine rice, almond milk, diced apple, and cinnamon in the Instant Pot
2. . Cook on high pressure for 6 minutes. Quick release.

CHOCOLATE BANANA OVERNIGHT OATS

Prep Time: 10 minutes Servings: 4

Nutrition per Serving: 200 calories, 6g protein, 35g carbohydrates, 5g fat, 6g fiber

Ingredients:

- 1 cup rolled oats
- 2 cups unsweetened almond milk
- 2 ripe bananas, mashed
- 2 tablespoons cocoa powder

Instructions:

1. Mix oats, almond milk, mashed bananas, and cocoa powder in the Instant Pot.
2. Refrigerate overnight. Stir before serving.

MAPLE PECAN QUINOA

Prep Time: 10 minutes Servings: 4

Nutrition per Serving: 200 calories, 5g protein, 35g carbohydrates, 5g fat, 4g fiber

Ingredients:

- 1 cup quinoa, rinsed
- 2 cups water
- 1/4 cup chopped pecans
- 2 tablespoons pure maple syrup

Instructions:

1. Combine quinoa, water, chopped pecans, and maple syrup in the Instant Pot.
2. Cook on high pressure for 1 minute. Allow a natural release.

BERRY QUINOA BREAKFAST BOWL

Prep Time: 10 minutes Servings: 4

Nutrition per Serving: 190 calories, 6g protein, 30g carbohydrates, 5g fat, 4g fiber

Ingredients:

- 1 cup quinoa, rinsed
- 2 cups water
- 1 cup mixed berries (fresh or frozen)
- 2 tablespoons slivered almonds

Instructions:

1. Combine quinoa, water, berries, and slivered almonds in the Instant Pot.
2. Cook on high pressure for 1 minute. Allow a natural release.

VEGGIE AND CHEESE EGG BITES

Prep Time: 15 minutes   Servings: 4

Nutrition per Serving: 140 calories, 10g protein, 5g carbohydrates, 8g fat, 1g fiber

Ingredients:

- 4 eggs
- 1/2 cup cottage cheese
- 1/2 cup diced bell peppers
- 1/4 cup shredded cheddar cheese

Instructions:

1. Blend eggs and cottage cheese.
2. Stir in bell peppers and cheddar cheese.
3. Pour into silicone molds.
4. Cook on high pressure for 8 minutes.

EGG WHITE AND SPINACH BREAKFAST BURRITOS

Prep Time: 15 minutes   Servings: 4

Nutrition per Serving: 180 calories, 15g protein, 15g carbohydrates, 8g fat, 2g fiber

Ingredients:

- 8 egg whites
- 2 cups fresh spinach, chopped
- 1/2 cup black beans, cooked
- 4 whole-wheat tortillas

Instructions:

Sauté spinach in the Instant Pot.

 Add egg whites and cook until set. Assemble burritos with spinach, egg whites, and black beans.

BERRY CHIA SEED JAM

Prep Time: 5 minutes (plus chilling time)

Servings: 8

Nutrition per Serving: 30 calories, 1g protein, 7g carbohydrates, 0g fat, 2g fiber

Ingredients:

- 2 cups mixed berries (strawberries, blueberries, raspberries)
- 2 tablespoons chia seeds
- 2 tablespoons honey

Instructions:

1. Blend berries, chia seeds, and honey in the Instant Pot.
2. Cook on sauté mode for 5 minutes.
3. Refrigerate until thickened.

SOUPS AND STEWS

VEGETABLE LENTIL SOUP

Preparation Time: 15 minutes Servings: 6

Nutrition per Serving: 150 calories, 25g carbohydrates, 5g fiber, 8g protein, 2g fat

Ingredients:

- 1 cup dry lentils, rinsed
- 4 cups vegetable broth
- 1 onion, diced
- 2 carrots, sliced
- 2 celery stalks, chopped
- 1 can diced tomatoes
- 2 cloves garlic, minced
- 1 tsp cumin
- 1 tsp paprika
- Salt and pepper to taste

Instructions:

1. Place all ingredients in the Instant Pot.
2. Set to high pressure for 10 minutes.
3. Allow a natural release for 5 minutes before venting.
4. Season with salt and pepper to taste.

CHICKEN AND QUINOA STEW

Preparation Time: 20 minutes Servings: 4

Nutrition per Serving: 220 calories, 20g carbohydrates, 3g fiber, 25g protein, 4g fat

Ingredients:

- 1 lb chicken breast, diced
- 1 cup quinoa, rinsed
- 4 cups chicken broth
- 1 onion, chopped
- 2 carrots, diced
- 2 cloves garlic, minced
- 1 tsp thyme
- Salt and pepper to taste

Instructions:

1. Combine all ingredients in the Instant Pot.
2. Set to high pressure for 8 minutes.
3. Allow a natural release for 10 minutes before venting.
4. Adjust seasoning as needed.

MINESTRONE SOUP

Preparation Time: 15 minutes Servings: 6

Nutrition per Serving: 180 calories, 30g carbohydrates, 5g fiber, 8g protein, 3g fat

Ingredients:

- 1 can kidney beans, drained and rinsed
- 1 cup diced zucchini
- 1 cup diced carrots
- 1 cup green beans, chopped
- 1 can diced tomatoes
- 1/2 cup whole wheat pasta
- 4 cups vegetable broth
- 1 tsp Italian seasoning
- Salt and pepper to taste

Instructions:

1. Combine all ingredients in the Instant Pot.
2. Set to high pressure for 6 minutes.
3. Allow a natural release for 5 minutes before venting.
4. Season with salt and pepper, and serve.

. BUTTERNUT SQUASH SOUP

Preparation Time: 20 minutes Servings: 4

Nutrition per Serving: 120 calories, 30g carbohydrates, 5g fiber, 2g protein, 1g fat

Ingredients:

- 1 medium butternut squash, peeled and diced
- 1 apple, peeled and diced
- 1 onion, chopped
- 2 cups vegetable broth
- 1 tsp cinnamon
- 1/2 tsp nutmeg
- Salt and pepper to taste

Instructions:

1. Combine all ingredients in the Instant Pot.
2. Set to high pressure for 8 minutes.
3. Allow a natural release for 5 minutes before venting.
4. Use an immersion blender to puree the soup.
5. Season with salt and pepper, and serve

TURKEY CHILI

Preparation Time: 25 minutes Servings: 5

Nutrition per Serving: 250 calories, 20g carbohydrates, 6g fiber, 25g protein, 8g fat

Ingredients:

- 1 lb ground turkey
- 1 can black beans, drained and rinsed
- 1 can diced tomatoes
- 1 onion, diced
- 2 cloves garlic, minced
- 2 tsp chili powder
- 1 tsp cumin
- Salt and pepper to taste

Instructions:

1. Brown turkey in Instant Pot using sauté function.
2. Add remaining ingredients.
3. Set to high pressure for 10 minutes.
4. Allow a natural release for 5 minutes before venting.

CHICKEN AND VEGETABLE STEW

Preparation Time: 15 minutes Servings: 4

Nutrition per Serving: 180 calories, 15g carbohydrates, 4g fiber, 20g protein, 5g fat

Ingredients:

- 1 lb chicken thighs, boneless and skinless
- 2 potatoes, diced
- 2 carrots, sliced
- 1 onion, chopped
- 2 cloves garlic, minced
- 4 cups chicken broth
- 1 tsp rosemary
- Salt and pepper to taste

Instructions:

1. Place all ingredients in the Instant Pot.
2. Set to high pressure for 10 minutes.
3. Allow a natural release for 5 minutes before venting.
4. Season with salt and pepper, and serve.

TOMATO BASIL SOUP

Preparation Time: 15 minutes Servings: 4

Nutrition per Serving: 120 calories, 15g carbohydrates, 3g fiber, 2g protein, 6g fat

Ingredients:

- 1 can crushed tomatoes
- 1 onion, chopped
- 2 cloves garlic, minced
- 4 cups vegetable broth
- 1/2 cup fresh basil, chopped
- 1 tsp oregano
- Salt and pepper to taste

Instructions:

1. Combine all ingredients in the Instant Pot.
2. Set to high pressure for 5 minutes.
3. Allow a natural release for 5 minutes before venting.
4. Use an immersion blender to blend the soup.
5. Season with salt and pepper, stir in fresh basil, and serve.

BLACK BEAN SOUP

Preparation Time: 20 minutes Servings: 6

Nutrition per Serving: 160 calories, 25g carbohydrates, 7g fiber, 8g protein, 2g fat

Ingredients:

- 2 cans black beans, drained and rinsed
- 1 onion, chopped
- 2 bell peppers, diced
- 2 cloves garlic, minced
- 4 cups vegetable broth
- 1 tsp cumin
- 1 tsp chili powder
- Salt and pepper to taste

Instructions:

1. Combine all ingredients in the Instant Pot.
2. Set to high pressure for 8 minutes.
3. Allow a natural release for 5 minutes before venting.
4. Season with salt and pepper, and serve

SWEET POTATO AND KALE STEW

Preparation Time: 15 minutes Servings: 4

Nutrition per Serving: 180 calories, 30g carbohydrates, 5g fiber, 5g protein, 4g fat

Ingredients:

- 2 sweet potatoes, peeled and diced
- 1 bunch kale, chopped
- 1 onion, chopped
- 2 cloves garlic, minced
- 4 cups vegetable broth
- 1 tsp thyme
- Salt and pepper to taste

Instructions:

1. Place all ingredients in the Instant Pot.
2. Set to high pressure for 8 minutes.
3. Allow a natural release for 5 minutes before venting.
4. Season with salt and pepper, and serve.

CHICKEN TORTILLA SOUP

Preparation Time: 20 minutes Servings: 5

Nutrition per Serving: 200 calories, 15g carbohydrates, 3g fiber, 20g protein, 6g fat

Ingredients:

- 1 lb chicken breasts, shredded
- 1 can black beans, drained and rinsed
- 1 can diced tomatoes
- 1 onion, chopped
- 2 cloves garlic, minced
- 4 cups chicken broth
- 1 tsp cumin
- 1 tsp chili powder
- Salt and pepper to taste

Instructions:

1. Combine all ingredients in the Instant Pot.
2. Set to high pressure for 8 minutes.
3. Allow a natural release for 5 minutes before venting.
4. Season with salt and pepper, and serve with tortilla strips

MUSHROOM BARLEY SOUP

Preparation Time: 20 minutes Servings: 6

Nutrition per Serving: 160 calories, 30g carbohydrates, 5g fiber, 6g protein, 2g fat

Ingredients:

- 1 cup pearl barley
- 8 oz mushrooms, sliced
- 1 onion, chopped
- 2 carrots, diced
- 2 cloves garlic, minced
- 4 cups vegetable broth
- 1 tsp thyme
- Salt and pepper to taste

Instructions:

1. Combine all ingredients in the Instant Pot.
2. Set to high pressure for 12 minutes.
3. Allow a natural release for 5 minutes before venting.
4. Season with salt and pepper, and serve.

SPLIT PEA SOUP

Preparation Time: 15 minutes Servings: 6

Nutrition per Serving: 180 calories, 30g carbohydrates, 10g fiber, 10g protein, 2g fat

Ingredients:

- 2 cups split peas, rinsed
- 1 ham hock
- 1 onion, chopped
- 2 carrots, diced
- 2 celery stalks, chopped
- 2 cloves garlic, minced
- 4 cups vegetable broth
- 1 tsp thyme
- Salt and pepper to taste

Instructions:

1. Place all ingredients in the Instant Pot.
2. Set to high pressure for 15 minutes.
3. Allow a natural release for 5 minutes before venting.
4. Remove ham hock, shred meat, and return to the soup.
5. Season with salt and pepper, and serve.

CABBAGE AND SAUSAGE STEW

Preparation Time: 15 minutes Servings: 4

Nutrition per Serving: 220 calories, 15g carbohydrates, 5g fiber, 12g protein, 14g fat

Ingredients:

- 1 lb turkey sausage, sliced
- 1 head cabbage, chopped
- 1 onion, chopped
- 2 cloves garlic, minced
- 4 cups chicken broth
- 1 tsp caraway seeds
- Salt and pepper to taste

Instructions:

1. Brown sausage in Instant Pot using sauté function.
2. Add remaining ingredients.
3. Set to high pressure for 8 minutes.
4. Allow a natural release for 5 minutes before venting.
5. Season with salt and pepper, and serve.

BEAN AND SPINACH STEW

Preparation Time: 15 minutes Servings: 4

Nutrition per Serving: 180 calories, 25g carbohydrates, 7g fiber, 10g protein, 5g fat

Ingredients:

- 2 cans white beans, drained and rinsed
- 1 onion, chopped
- 2 carrots, diced
- 2 cloves garlic, minced
- 4 cups vegetable broth
- 2 cups spinach, chopped
- 1 tsp Italian seasoning
- Salt and pepper to taste

Instructions:

1. Combine all ingredients in the Instant Pot.
2. Set to high pressure for 8 minutes.
3. Allow a natural release for 5 minutes before venting.
4. Stir in chopped spinach until wilted.
5. Season with salt and pepper, and serve.

SHRIMP AND VEGETABLE CURRY SOUP

Preparation Time: 20 minutes Servings: 4

Nutrition per Serving: 230 calories, 20g carbohydrates, 4g fiber, 15g protein, 10g fat

Ingredients:

- 1 lb shrimp, peeled and deveined
- 1 can coconut milk
- 1 onion, chopped
- 1 bell pepper, sliced
- 1 zucchini, diced
- 2 cloves garlic, minced
- 2 tbsp red curry paste
- 4 cups chicken broth
- Salt and pepper to taste

Instructions:

1. Combine all ingredients in the Instant Pot, except shrimp.
2. Set to high pressure for 5 minutes.
3. Allow a natural release for 5 minutes before venting.
4. Stir in shrimp until cooked.
5. Season with salt and pepper, and serve.

LEMON CHICKEN ORZO SOUP

Preparation Time: 15 minutes Servings: 4

Nutrition per Serving: 200 calories, 20g carbohydrates, 2g fiber, 20g protein, 4g fat

Ingredients:

- 1 lb chicken breasts, diced
- 1 cup orzo pasta
- 1 lemon, juiced and zested
- 1 carrot, sliced
- 2 celery stalks, chopped
- 2 cloves garlic, minced
- 4 cups chicken broth
- 1 tsp thyme
- Salt and pepper to taste

Instructions:

1. Combine all ingredients in the Instant Pot.
2. Set to high pressure for 8 minutes.
3. Allow a natural release for 5 minutes before venting.
4. Season with salt and pepper, and serve.

. TURKEY AND VEGETABLE QUINOA STEW

Preparation Time: 20 minutes Servings: 4

Nutrition per Serving: 220 calories, 25g carbohydrates, 5g fiber, 20g protein, 4g fat

Ingredients:

- 1 lb ground turkey
- 1 cup quinoa, rinsed
- 2 carrots, diced
- 1 bell pepper, chopped
- 1 onion, chopped
- 2 cloves garlic, minced
- 4 cups chicken broth
- 1 tsp cumin
- 1 tsp paprika
- Salt and pepper to taste

Instructions:

1. Brown turkey in Instant Pot using sauté function.
2. Add remaining ingredients.
3. Set to high pressure for 8 minutes.
4. Allow a natural release for 5 minutes before venting.
5. Adjust seasoning and serve.

ITALIAN WEDDING SOUP

Preparation Time: 20 minutes Servings: 6

Nutrition per Serving: 160 calories, 15g carbohydrates, 3g fiber, 18g protein, 4g fat

Ingredients:

- 1/2 lb lean ground turkey
- 1/2 cup whole wheat breadcrumbs
- 1 egg, beaten
- 1 onion, chopped
- 2 carrots, sliced
- 2 celery stalks, chopped
- 2 cloves garlic, minced
- 4 cups chicken broth
- 1 cup spinach, chopped
- Salt and pepper to taste

Instructions:

1. In a bowl, combine ground turkey, breadcrumbs, and beaten egg. Form into small meatballs.
2. Brown meatballs in Instant Pot using sauté function.
3. Add remaining ingredients.
4. Set to high pressure for 5 minutes.
5. Allow a natural release for 5 minutes before venting.
6. Season with salt and pepper, and serve.

MOROCCAN CHICKPEA STEW

Preparation Time: 20 minutes Servings: 4

Nutrition per Serving: 200 calories, 30g carbohydrates, 7g fiber, 8g protein, 5g fat

Ingredients:

- 2 cans chickpeas, drained and rinsed
- 1 onion, chopped
- 2 carrots, diced
- 1 zucchini, chopped
- 2 cloves garlic, minced
- 1 can diced tomatoes
- 4 cups vegetable broth
- 1 tsp cumin
- 1 tsp coriander
- Salt and pepper to taste

Instructions:

1. Combine all ingredients in the Instant Pot.
2. Set to high pressure for 10 minutes.
3. Allow a natural release for 5 minutes before venting.
4. Season with salt and pepper, and serve.

CAULIFLOWER AND BROCCOLI SOUP

Preparation Time: 15 minutes Servings: 4

Nutrition per Serving: 120 calories, 15g carbohydrates, 5g fiber, 5g protein, 5g fat

Ingredients:

- 1 head cauliflower, chopped
- 2 cups broccoli florets
- 1 onion, chopped
- 2 cloves garlic, minced
- 4 cups vegetable broth
- 1/2 cup low-fat milk
- 1 tsp nutmeg
- Salt and pepper to taste

Instructions:

1. Combine cauliflower, broccoli, onion, garlic, and vegetable broth in the Instant Pot.
2. Set to high pressure for 8 minutes.
3. Use an immersion blender to puree the soup.
4. Stir in milk, nutmeg, salt, and pepper.
5. Adjust seasoning and serve.

QUINOA AND BLACK BEAN CHILI

Preparation Time: 25 minutes Servings: 6

Nutrition per Serving: 250 calories, 30g carbohydrates, 8g fiber, 12g protein, 6g fat

Ingredients:

- 1 cup quinoa, rinsed
- 2 cans black beans, drained and rinsed
- 1 onion, chopped
- 1 bell pepper, diced
- 2 cloves garlic, minced
- 1 can diced tomatoes
- 4 cups vegetable broth
- 2 tsp chili powder
- Salt and pepper to taste

Instructions:

1. Combine all ingredients in the Instant Pot.
2. Set to high pressure for 10 minutes.
3. Allow a natural release for 5 minutes before venting.
4. Season with salt and pepper, and serve.

RED LENTIL AND SPINACH SOUP

Preparation Time: 15 minutes Servings: 4

Nutrition per Serving: 160 calories, 20g carbohydrates, 5g fiber, 10g protein, 3g fat

Ingredients:

- 1 cup red lentils, rinsed
- 2 cups spinach, chopped
- 2 carrots, diced
- 2 cloves garlic, minced
- 4 cups vegetable broth
- 1 tsp cumin
- 1 tsp turmeric
- Salt and pepper to taste

Instructions:

1. Combine all ingredients in the Instant Pot.
2. Set to high pressure for 6 minutes.
3. Allow a natural release for 5 minutes before venting.
4. Season with salt and pepper, and serve.

TUSCAN WHITE BEAN AND KALE SOUP

Preparation Time: 20 minutes Servings: 4

Nutrition per Serving: 180 calories, 25g carbohydrates, 5g fiber, 10g protein, 4g fat

Ingredients:

- 2 cans white beans, drained and rinsed
- 1 bunch kale, chopped
- 1 onion, chopped
- 2 carrots, diced
- 2 cloves garlic, minced
- 4 cups vegetable broth
- 1 tsp rosemary
- Salt and pepper to taste

Instructions:

1. Combine all ingredients in the Instant Pot.
2. Set to high pressure for 8 minutes.
3. Allow a natural release for 5 minutes before venting.
4. Season with salt and pepper, and serve

BROCCOLI AND CHEDDAR SOUP

Preparation Time: 20 minute Servings: 4

Nutrition per Serving: 180 calories, 20g carbohydrates, 4g fiber, 8g protein, 8g fat

Ingredients:

- 2 cups broccoli florets
- 1 onion, chopped
- 2 cloves garlic, minced
- 4 cups vegetable broth
- 1 cup lowfat milk
- 1 cup sharp cheddar cheese, shredded
- Salt and pepper to taste

Instructions:

1. Combine broccoli, onion, garlic, and vegetable broth in the Instant Pot.
2. Set to high pressure for 8 minutes.
3. Use an immersion blender to puree the soup.
4. Stir in milk and cheddar cheese until melted.
5. Season with salt and pepper, and serve.

CHICKEN AND RICE SOUP

Preparation Time: 20 minutes Servings: 4

Nutrition per Serving: 220 calories, 25g carbohydrates, 2g fiber, 20g protein, 4g fat

Ingredients:

- 1 lb chicken thighs, boneless and skinless
- 1 cup white rice, rinsed
- 2 carrots, sliced
- 2 celery stalks, chopped
- 1 onion, chopped
- 2 cloves garlic, minced
- 4 cups chicken broth
- 1 tsp thyme
- Salt and pepper to taste

Instructions:

1. Place all ingredients in the Instant Pot.
2. Set to high pressure for 10 minutes.
3. Allow a natural release for 5 minutes before venting.
4. Shred chicken, season with salt and pepper, and serve.

POULTRY DISHES

LEMON GARLIC CHICKEN

Preparation Time: 15 minutes Servings: 4

Nutrition per Serving: Calories: 250, Carbs: 5g, Protein: 30g, Fat: 12g

Ingredients:

- 4 boneless, skinless chicken breasts
- 1/4 cup olive oil
- 3 cloves garlic, minced
- Juice of 1 lemon
- 1 teaspoon dried oregano

Instructions:

1. Sauté garlic in olive oil, add chicken, lemon juice, and oregano
2. Pressure cook for 10 minutes.

TURKEY CHILI

Preparation Time: 25 minutes Servings: 6

Nutrition per Serving: Calories: 280, Carbs: 22g, Protein: 30g, Fat: 8g

Ingredients:

- 1 lb ground turkey
- 1 can (15 oz) low sodium kidney beans, drained
- 1 can (15 oz) diced tomatoes
- 1 onion, diced
- 2 tablespoons chili powder

Instructions:

1. Sauté turkey and onions, add beans, tomatoes, and chili powder.
2. Pressure cook for 15 minutes.

CHICKEN AND VEGETABLE STIRFRY

Preparation Time: 20 minutes Servings: 4

Nutrition per Serving: Calories: 180, Carbs: 12g, Protein: 25g, Fat: 5g

Ingredients:

- 1 lb boneless, skinless chicken thighs, sliced
- 2 cups broccoli florets
- 1 bell pepper, sliced
- 3 tablespoons low sodium soy sauce
- 1 tablespoon sesame oil

Instructions:

1. Sauté chicken, add vegetables, soy sauce, and sesame oil.
2. Pressure cook for 5 minutes.

CHICKEN AND QUINOA CASSEROLE

Preparation Time: 30 minutes Servings: 4

Nutrition per Serving: Calories: 320, Carbs: 25g, Protein: 28g, Fat: 12g

Ingredients:

- 1 lb. boneless, skinless chicken breasts
- 1 cup quinoa, rinsed
- 2 cups low sodium chicken broth
- 1 cup mixed vegetables (peas, carrots, corn)

Instructions:

1. Place chicken, quinoa, broth, and vegetables in Instant Pot.
2. Pressure cook for 15 minutes.

CHICKEN AND BROCCOLI

Preparation Time: 20 minutes Servings: 4

Nutrition per Serving: Calories: 220, Carbs: 10g, Protein: 26g, Fat: 8g

Ingredients:

- 1.5 lbs boneless, skinless chicken thighs, sliced
- 2 cups broccoli florets
- 3 tablespoons low sodium soy sauce
- 1 tablespoon rice vinegar

Instructions:

1. Sauté chicken, add broccoli, soy sauce, and rice vinegar.
2. Pressure cook for 8 minutes.

HERB CHICKEN THIGHS

Preparation Time: 15 minute Servings: 4

Nutrition per Serving: Calories: 260, Carbs: 2g, Protein: 30g, Fat: 14g

Ingredients:

- 1.5 lbs. bone in, skin on chicken thighs
- 3 cloves garlic, minced
- 1 teaspoon dried thyme
- 1 teaspoon dried rosemary

Instructions:

1. Rub chicken with garlic, thyme, and rosemary.
2. Pressure cook for 12 minutes.

BBQ CHICKEN

Preparation Time: 15 minutes Servings: 4

Nutrition per Serving: Calories: 280, Carbs: 15g, Protein: 28g, Fat: 12g

Ingredients:

- 2 lbs. boneless, skinless chicken breasts
- 1 cup sugar free barbecue sauce
- 1 teaspoon smoked paprika
- 1/2 teaspoon garlic powder

Instructions:

1. Coat chicken with BBQ sauce, paprika, and garlic powder.
2. Pressure cook for 15 minutes.

CHICKEN AND MUSHROOM SKILLET

Preparation Time: 25 minutes Servings: 4

Nutrition per Serving: Calories: 230, Carbs: 8g, Protein: 28g, Fat: 10g

Ingredients:

- 1.5 lbs. boneless, skinless chicken breasts
- 2 cups sliced mushrooms
- 1 onion, diced
- 1/2 cup low sodium chicken broth

Instructions:

1. Sauté chicken, mushrooms, and onions.
2. Add chicken broth.
3. Pressure cook for 10 minutes.

LEMON HERB TURKEY BREAST

Preparation Time: 15 minutes Servings: 6

Nutrition per Serving: Calories: 180, Carbs: 2g, Protein: 25g, Fat: 8g

Ingredients:

- 3 lbs boneless, skinless turkey breast
- Juice of 2 lemons
- 1 teaspoon dried thyme
- 1 teaspoon dried sage

Instructions:

1. Rub turkey with lemon juice, thyme, and sage.
2. Pressure cook for 25 minutes.

TERIYAKI CHICKEN

Preparation Time: 20 minutes Servings: 4

Nutrition per Serving: Calories: 250, Carbs: 20g, Protein: 26g, Fat: 8g

Ingredients:

1.5 lbs. boneless, skinless chicken thighs, sliced

1/2 cup low sodium soy sauce

1/4 cup honey or sugar substitute

2 cloves garlic, minced

Instructions:

1. Combine chicken, soy sauce, honey, and garlic.
2. Pressure cook for 12 minutes.

CHICKEN PICCATA

Preparation Time: 20 minutes Servings: 4

Nutrition per Serving: Calories: 280, Carbs: 10g, Protein: 30g, Fat: 12g

Ingredients:

- 1.5 lbs chicken cutlets
- 1/2 cup chicken broth
- Juice of 1 lemon
- 2 tablespoons capers

Instructions:

1. Sauté chicken, add broth, lemon juice, and capers.
2. Pressure cook for 8 minutes.

ORANGE GINGER CHICKEN

Preparation Time: 15 minutes Servings: 4

Nutrition per Serving: Calories: 240, Carbs: 12g, Protein: 26g, Fat: 10g

Ingredients:

- 1.5 lbs boneless, skinless chicken breasts
- Juice of 2 oranges
- 1 tablespoon grated ginger
- 2 tablespoons low sodium soy sauce

Instructions:

1. Combine chicken, orange juice, ginger, and soy sauce.
2. Pressure cook for 12 minutes.

CHICKEN AND BROWN RICE

Preparation Time: 30 minutes Servings: 4

Nutrition per Serving: Calories: 290, Carbs: 25g, Protein: 28g, Fat: 8g

Ingredients:

- 1.5 lbs. boneless, skinless chicken thighs, sliced
- 1 cup brown rice
- 2 cups low sodium chicken broth
- 1 cup mixed vegetables (peas, carrots, corn)

Instructions:

1. Place chicken, rice, broth, and vegetables in Instant Pot.
2. Pressure cook for 15 minutes.

CHICKEN AND SPINACH CURRY

Preparation Time: 25 minutes Servings: 4

Nutrition per Serving: Calories: 220, Carbs: 8g, Protein: 28g, Fat: 8g

Ingredients:

- 1.5 lbs. boneless, skinless chicken thighs, diced
- 2 cups fresh spinach
- 1 can (14 oz) coconut milk
- 2 tablespoons curry powder

Instructions:

1. Sauté chicken, add spinach, coconut milk, and curry powder.
2. Pressure cook for 10 minutes.

ROSEMARY BALSAMIC CHICKEN

Preparation Time: 20 minutes Servings: 4

Nutrition per Serving: Calories: 260, Carbs: 8g, Protein: 30g, Fat: 12g

Ingredients:

- 1.5 lbs. bone in, skin on chicken thighs
- 1/4 cup balsamic vinegar
- 2 tablespoons olive oil
- 1 teaspoon dried rosemary

Instructions:

1. Mix chicken with balsamic vinegar, olive oil, and rosemary.
2. Pressure cook for 12 minutes.

CHICKEN AND BLACK BEAN STEW

Preparation Time: 25 minutes Servings: 6

Nutrition per Serving: Calories: 230, Carbs: 20g, Protein: 26g, Fat: 6g

Ingredients:

- 1.5 lbs boneless, skinless chicken breasts
- 1 can (15 oz) black beans, drained
- 1 can (14 oz) diced tomatoes
- 1 onion, diced
- 2 teaspoons cumin

Instructions:

- Sauté chicken and onions, add black beans, tomatoes, and cumin.
- Pressure cook for 15 minutes.

CHICKEN AND ASPARAGUS

Preparation Time: 20 minutes Servings: 4

Nutrition per Serving: Calories: 200, Carbs: 8g, Protein: 28g, Fat: 6g

Ingredients:

- 1.5 lbs boneless, skinless chicken breasts
- 1 bunch asparagus, trimmed
- 1 lemon, sliced
- 2 tablespoons olive oil

Instructions:

1. Sauté chicken, add asparagus, lemon slices, and olive oil.
2. Pressure cook for 8 minutes.

CHICKEN AND VEGETABLE CURRY

Preparation Time: 25 minutes Servings: 4

Nutrition per Serving: Calories: 240, Carbs: 15g, Protein: 26g, Fat: 10g

Ingredients:

- 1.5 lbs. boneless, skinless chicken thighs, diced
- 2 cups mixed vegetables (bell peppers, zucchini, carrots)
- 1 can (14 oz) coconut milk
- 2 tablespoons curry paste

Instructions:

1. Sauté chicken, add vegetables, coconut milk, and curry paste.
2. Pressure cook for 10 minutes.

GREEK CHICKEN SALAD

Preparation Time: 20 minutes Servings: 4

Nutrition per Serving: Calories: 280, Carbs: 10g, Protein: 28g, Fat: 14g

Ingredients:

- 1.5 lbs. boneless, skinless chicken breasts
- 2 cups cherry tomatoes, halved
- 1 cucumber, diced
- 1/2 cup feta cheese, crumbled
- 2 tablespoons olive oil

Instructions:

1. Sauté chicken, mix with tomatoes, cucumber, feta, and olive oil.
2. Pressure cook for 8 minutes.

CHICKEN AND CAULIFLOWER RICE

Preparation Time: 20 minutes Servings: 4

Nutrition per Serving: Calories: 220, Carbs: 10g, Protein: 28g, Fat: 8g

Ingredients:

- 1.5 lbs. boneless, skinless chicken breasts
- 1 head cauliflower, riced
- 1 cup chicken broth
- 2 cloves garlic, minced

Instructions:

- Sauté chicken and garlic, add cauliflower rice and broth.
- Pressure cook for 8 minutes.

PESTO CHICKEN

Preparation Time: 15 minutes Servings: 4

Nutrition per Serving: Calories: 260, Carbs: 5g, Protein: 30g, Fat: 14g

Ingredients:

- 1.5 lbs. boneless, skinless chicken thighs
- 1/2 cup basil pesto
- 1/4 cup grated Parmesan cheese
- 1/2 cup cherry tomatoes, halved

Instructions:

1. Coat chicken with pesto, sprinkle with Parmesan, add tomatoes.
2. Pressure cook for 12 minutes.

CHICKEN AND SWEET POTATO STEW

Preparation Time: 25 minutes Servings: 6

Nutrition per Serving: Calories: 260, Carbs: 20g, Protein: 28g, Fat: 8g

Ingredients:

- 1.5 lbs. boneless, skinless chicken thighs, diced
- 2 sweet potatoes, peeled and cubed
- 1 can (14 oz.) diced tomatoes
- 1 onion, diced
- 2 teaspoons paprika

Instructions:

1. Sauté chicken and onions, add sweet potatoes, tomatoes, and paprika.
2. Pressure cook for 15 minutes.

CHICKEN AND LENTIL SOUP

Preparation Time: 30 minutes Servings: 6

Nutrition per Serving: Calories: 240, Carbs: 25g, Protein: 26g, Fat: 6g

Ingredients:

- 1.5 lbs. boneless, skinless chicken breasts
- 1 cup dried green lentils, rinsed
- 2 carrots, diced
- 1 onion, diced
- 1 teaspoon cumin

Instructions:

1. Sauté chicken and onions, add lentils, carrots, and cumin.
2. Pressure cook for 15 minutes.

CHICKEN AND CABBAGE STIR-FRY

Preparation Time: 20 minutes Servings: 4

Nutrition per Serving: Calories: 200, Carbs: 15g, Protein: 26g, Fat: 8g

Ingredients:

- 1.5 lbs. boneless, skinless chicken thighs, sliced
- 4 cups shredded cabbage
- 1 bell pepper, sliced
- 3 tablespoons low sodium soy sauce

Instructions:

1. Sauté chicken, add cabbage, bell pepper, and soy sauce.
2. Pressure cook for 5 minutes.

CHICKEN AND AVOCADO SALAD

Preparation Time: 15 minutes Servings: 4

Nutrition per Serving: Calories: 280, Carbs: 10g, Protein: 28g, Fat: 14g

Ingredients:

- 1.5 lbs. boneless, skinless chicken breasts
- 2 avocados, diced
- 1 cup cherry tomatoes, halved
- 1/4 cup cilantro, chopped

Instructions:

1. Sauté chicken, mix with avocados, tomatoes, and cilantro.
2. Pressure cook for 8 minutes.

SEA FOOD AND FISH DIET

LEMON GARLIC SHRIMP

Preparation Time: 15 minutes Servings: 4

Nutrition per Serving: Calories: 180 Carbohydrates: 4g Protein: 20g Fat: 9g

Ingredients:

- 1 lb. shrimp, peeled and deveined
- 2 tbsp. olive oil
- 3 cloves garlic, minced
- 1 lemon (zest and juice)
- 1 tsp dried oregano
- Salt and pepper to taste

Instructions:

1. Set Instant Pot to sauté mode, add olive oil, and sauté garlic until fragrant.
2. Add shrimp, lemon zest, lemon juice, oregano, salt, and pepper. Stir well.
3. Close the lid, set to high pressure for 2 minutes, then quick release.

TILAPIA WITH TOMATO AND BASIL:

Preparation Time: 15 minutes Servings: 4

Nutrition per Serving: Calories: 180 Carbohydrates: 6g Protein: 22g Fat: 7g

Ingredients:

- 4 tilapia fillets
- 1 cup cherry tomatoes, halved
- 2 tbsp. olive oil
- 2 tbsp. fresh basil, chopped
- Garlic powder, salt, and pepper to taste

Instructions:

1. Season tilapia with garlic powder, salt, and pepper.
2. Place tilapia in Instant Pot, top with tomatoes, basil, and olive oil.
3. Set to high pressure for 4 minutes, then quick release

SALMON WITH DILL SAUCE

Preparation Time: 20 minutes Servings: 3

Nutrition per Serving: Calories: 250 Carbohydrates: 5g Protein: 25g Fat: 14g

Ingredients:

- 3 salmon fillets
- 1 cup chicken or vegetable broth
- 2 tbsp. fresh dill, chopped
- 1 tbsp. Dijon mustard
- Salt and pepper to taste

Instructions:

1. Place broth in the Instant Pot, add salmon fillets.
2. Set to high pressure for 3 minutes, then quick release.
3. In a separate bowl, mix dill, mustard, salt, and pepper. Spoon over salmon.

GARLIC BUTTER SCALLOPS

Preparation Time: 10 minutes Servings: 2

Nutrition per Serving: Calories: 220 Carbohydrates: 3g Protein: 18g Fat: 15g

Ingredients:

- 1 lb. scallops
- 3 tbsp. unsalted butter
- 4 cloves garlic, minced
- 2 tbsp. fresh parsley, chopped
- Salt and pepper to taste

Instructions:

1. Set Instant Pot to sauté mode, melt butter, add garlic, and sauté.
2. Add scallops, season with salt and pepper, cook for 23 minutes per side.
3. Sprinkle with parsley before serving.

LIME CILANTRO COD

Preparation Time: 15 minutes Servings: 3

Nutrition per Serving: Calories: 160 Carbohydrates: 2g Protein: 22g Fat: 7g

Ingredients:

- 3 cod fillets
- 1 lime (zest and juice)
- 2 tbsp fresh cilantro, chopped
- 1 tbsp olive oil
- Salt and pepper to taste

Instructions:

1. Rub cod with olive oil, lime zest, lime juice, cilantro, salt, and pepper.
2. Place cod in Instant Pot, set to high pressure for 4 minutes, then quick release.
3. Spoon cooking juices over the cod before serving.

SHRIMP AND BROCCOLI STIR-FRY

Preparation Time: 20 minutes Servings: 4

Nutrition per Serving: Calories: 200 Carbohydrates: 8g Protein: 24g Fat: 8g

Ingredients:

- 1 lb. shrimp, peeled and deveined
- 2 cups broccoli florets
- 2 tbsp. low sodium soy sauce
- 1 tbsp. sesame oil
- 1 tsp ginger, grated
- 2 cloves garlic, minced

Instructions:

1. Set Instant Pot to sauté mode, add sesame oil, ginger, and garlic.
2. Add shrimp and broccoli, stir in soy sauce.
3. Close the lid, set to high pressure for 1 minute, then quick release.

MEDITERRANEAN FISH STEW

Preparation Time: 25 minutes Servings: 6

Nutrition per Serving: Calories: 210 Carbohydrates: 12g Protein: 20g Fat: 9g

Ingredients:

- 1 lb. white fish fillets (e.g., cod or haddock)
- 1 can (14 oz.) diced tomatoes, drained
- 1 onion, diced
- 2 cloves garlic, minced
- 1 cup low sodium chicken broth
- 1 tsp dried oregano
- 1 tsp dried basil
- Salt and pepper to taste

Instructions:

1. Set Instant Pot to sauté mode, sauté onions and garlic until softened.
2. Add tomatoes, chicken broth, oregano, basil, salt, and pepper.
3. Add fish fillets, close the lid, set to high pressure for 3 minutes, then quick release.

COCONUT CURRY SHRIMP:

Preparation Time: 25 minutes Servings: 4

Nutrition per Serving: Calories: 230 Carbohydrates: 8g Protein: 20g Fat: 14g

Ingredients:

- 1 lb. shrimp, peeled and deveined
- 1 can (14 oz.) coconut milk
- 2 tbsp. red curry paste
- 1 bell pepper, sliced
- 1 zucchini, sliced
- 1 tbsp. fish sauce
- Fresh cilantro for garnish

Instructions:

1. Set Instant Pot to sauté mode, combine coconut milk and red curry paste.
2. Add shrimp, bell pepper, zucchini, and fish sauce. Stir well.
3. Close the lid, set to high pressure for 2 minutes, then quick release. Garnish with cilantro.

CAJUN SPICED CATFISH

Preparation Time: 20 minutes Servings: 4

Nutrition per Serving: Calories: 180 Carbohydrates: 5g Protein: 22g Fat: 8g

Ingredients:

- 4 catfish fillets
- 1 tbsp. Cajun seasoning
- 1 tbsp. olive oil
- 1 lemon, sliced
- Salt and pepper to taste

Instructions:

1. Rub catfish fillets with Cajun seasoning, salt, and pepper.
2. Set Instant Pot to sauté mode, add olive oil, and sear catfish on both sides.
3. Place lemon slices on top, close the lid, set to high pressure for 4 minutes, then quick release.

LEMON HERB MAHI-MAHI

Preparation Time: 15 minutes Servings: 2

Nutrition per Serving: Calories: 220 Carbohydrates: 3g Protein: 28g Fat: 10g

Ingredients:

- 2 mahi-mahi fillets
- 1 lemon (zest and juice)
- 2 tbsp. fresh parsley, chopped
- 1 tbsp. olive oil
- 1 tsp dried thyme
- Salt and pepper to taste

Instructions:

1. Rub mahi-mahi with olive oil, lemon zest, lemon juice, parsley, thyme, salt, and pepper.
2. Place fillets in Instant Pot, set to high pressure for 3 minutes, then quick release

LEMON HERB TUNA STEAKS

Preparation Time: 20 minutes Servings: 2

Nutrition per Serving: Calories: 250 Carbohydrates: 5g Protein: 30g Fat: 12g

Ingredients:

- 2 tuna steaks
- 1 lemon (zest and juice)
- 2 tbsp fresh dill, chopped
- 1 tbsp olive oil
- 1 tsp dried rosemary
- Salt and pepper to taste

Instructions:

1. Rub tuna steaks with olive oil, lemon zest, lemon juice, dill, rosemary, salt, and pepper.
2. Place steaks in Instant Pot, set to high pressure for 3 minutes, then quick release.

SHRIMP AND ASPARAGUS RISOTTO

Preparation Time: 25 minutes Servings: 4

Nutrition per Serving: Calories: 280 Carbohydrates: 30g Protein: 18g Fat: 10g

Ingredients:

- 1 lb. shrimp, peeled and deveined
- 1 cup Arborio rice
- 2 cups asparagus, chopped
- 4 cups low sodium chicken broth
- 1/2 cup dry white wine
- 1/2 cup Parmesan cheese, grated
- 2 tbsp. olive oil
- 1 onion, diced
- 2 cloves garlic, minced
- Salt and pepper to taste

Instructions:

1. Set Instant Pot to sauté mode, sauté onion and garlic in olive oil.
2. Add Arborio rice, stir until lightly toasted. Pour in white wine and let it evaporate.
3. Add shrimp, asparagus, and chicken broth. Close the lid, set to high pressure for 5 minutes, then quick release. Stir in Parmesan before serving.

HERB CRUSTED HADDOCK

Preparation Time: 20 minutes Servings: 3

Nutrition per Serving: Calories: 190 Carbohydrates: 2g Protein: 25g Fat: 9g

Ingredients:

- 3 haddock fillets
- 2 tbsp. fresh parsley, chopped
- 1 tbsp. fresh thyme, chopped
- 1 tbsp. olive oil
- 1 lemon, sliced
- Salt and pepper to taste

Instructions:

1. Mix parsley, thyme, olive oil, salt, and pepper. Rub the mixture onto haddock fillets.
2. Place fillets in Instant Pot, add lemon slices on top. Set to high pressure for 4 minutes, then quick release.

CILANTRO LIME SHRIMP TACOS

Preparation Time: 20 minutes Servings: 4

Nutrition per Serving: Calories: 220 Carbohydrates: 15g Protein: 20g Fat: 10g

Ingredients:

- 1 lb. shrimp, peeled and deveined
- 1/4 cup fresh cilantro, chopped
- 2 limes (zest and juice)
- 1 tbsp. olive oil
- 1 tsp ground cumin
- 1 tsp chili powder
- Salt and pepper to taste
- Whole wheat tortillas

Instructions:

1. Set Instant Pot to sauté mode, sauté shrimp in olive oil, cumin, and chili powder.
2. Add cilantro, lime zest, and lime juice. Stir well.
3. Serve in whole wheat tortillas.

SPICY GARLIC MUSSELS

Preparation Time: 15 minutes Servings: 2

Nutrition per Serving: Calories: 180 Carbohydrates: 7g Protein: 15g Fat: 8g

Ingredients:

- 2 lbs. mussels, cleaned and DE bearded
- 3 cloves garlic, minced
- 1/2 cup white wine
- 2 tbsp. tomato paste
- 1 tbsp. olive oil
- 1 tsp red pepper flakes
- Fresh parsley for garnish

Instructions:

1. Set Instant Pot to sauté mode, sauté garlic in olive oil.
2. Add white wine, tomato paste, red pepper flakes, and mussels. Close the lid, set to high pressure for 2 minutes, then quick release. Garnish with fresh parsley.

SESAME GINGER SALMON

Preparation Time: 25 minutes Servings: 2

Nutrition per Serving: Calories: 280 Carbohydrates: 10g Protein: 28g Fat: 15g

Ingredients:

- 2 salmon fillets
- 2 tbsp. low sodium soy sauce
- 1 tbsp. sesame oil
- 1 tbsp. rice vinegar
- 1 tbsp. fresh ginger, grated
- 1 tbsp. sesame seeds
- Green onions for garnish

Instructions:

1. Mix soy sauce, sesame oil, rice vinegar, and ginger. Marinate salmon in the mixture.
2. Place salmon in Instant Pot, sprinkle with sesame seeds.
3. Set to high pressure for 3 minutes, then quick release. Garnish with green onions.

GARLIC PARMESAN SHRIMP PASTA

Preparation Time: 25 minutes Servings: 4

Nutrition per Serving: Calories: 320 Carbohydrates: 30g Protein: 25g Fat: 12g

Ingredients:

- 1 lb shrimp, peeled and deveined
- 8 oz whole wheat spaghetti
- 3 cups low sodium chicken broth
- 4 cloves garlic, minced
- 1/2 cup Parmesan cheese, grated
- 2 tbsp. olive oil
- Fresh parsley for garnish

Instructions:

1. Set Instant Pot to sauté mode, sauté garlic in olive oil.
2. Add shrimp, cook for 23 minutes. Add spaghetti and chicken broth.
3. Close the lid, set to high pressure for pasta cooking time (check pasta package instructions), then quick release. Stir in Parmesan, garnish with parsley.

TUNA AND WHITE BEAN SALAD

Preparation Time: 20 minutes Servings: 4

Nutrition per Serving: Calories: 240 Carbohydrates: 20g Protein: 22g Fat: 10g

Ingredients:

- 2 cans (5 oz each) tuna, drained
- 2 cans (15 oz each) cannellini beans, drained and rinsed
- 1 red onion, finely chopped
- 1/4 cup fresh parsley, chopped
- 2 tbsp red wine vinegar
- 2 tbsp olive oil
- Salt and pepper to taste

Instructions:

1. Combine tuna, beans, red onion, and parsley in Instant Pot.
2. In a small bowl, whisk together red wine vinegar, olive oil, salt, and pepper. Pour over the tuna mixture.
3. Gently toss, set Instant Pot to sauté mode for a few minutes to warm the salad

SHRIMP AND ZUCCHINI NOODLES

Preparation Time: 15 minutes Servings: 3

Nutrition per Serving: Calories: 180 Carbohydrates: 6g Protein: 22g Fat: 8g

Ingredients:

- 1 lb. shrimp, peeled and deveined
- 3 zucchinis, spiralizer
- 2 tbsp. olive oil
- 3 cloves garlic, minced
- 1 tsp red pepper flakes
- 1 lemon (zest and juice)
- Salt and pepper to taste

Instructions:

1. Set Instant Pot to sauté mode, sauté garlic in olive oil.
2. Add shrimp, zucchini noodles, red pepper flakes, lemon zest, and lemon juice. Stir well.
3. Close the lid, set to high pressure for 2 minutes, then quick release.

LEMON DILL TUNA SALAD

Preparation Time: 15 minutes Servings: 4

Nutrition per Serving: Calories: 180 Carbohydrates: 5g Protein: 20g Fat: 9g

Ingredients:

- 2 cans (5 oz each) tuna, drained
- 1/2 cup Greek yogurt
- 2 tbsp. fresh dill, chopped
- 1 lemon (zest and juice)
- 1 celery stalk, finely chopped
- Salt and pepper to taste

Instructions:

1. In a bowl, combine tuna, Greek yogurt, dill, lemon zest, lemon juice, celery, salt, and pepper.
2. Mix well and serve. Enjoy on whole wheat crackers or as a salad.

MISO GLAZED COD

Preparation Time: 20 minute   Servings: 2

Nutrition per Serving: Calories: 230 Carbohydrates: 10g Protein: 28g Fat: 8g

Ingredients:

- 2 cod fillets
- 2 tbsp. white miso paste
- 1 tbsp. low sodium soy sauce
- 1 tbsp. rice vinegar
- 1 tbsp. honey
- 1 tsp sesame oil
- 1 tsp fresh ginger, grated
- Green onions for garnish

Instructions:

1. In a bowl, whisk together miso paste, soy sauce, rice vinegar, honey, sesame oil, and ginger.
2. Brush the mixture over cod fillets.
3. Place fillets in Instant Pot, set to high pressure for 4 minutes, then quick release. Garnish with green onions.

MEDITERRANEAN TUNA QUINOA BOWL

Preparation Time: 25 minutes Servings: 4

Nutrition per Serving: Calories: 280 Carbohydrates: 30g Protein: 20g Fat: 10g

Ingredients:

- 2 cups cooked quinoa
- 2 cans (5 oz each) tuna, drained
- 1 cup cherry tomatoes, halved
- 1 cucumber, diced
- 1/2 cup Kalamata olives, sliced
- 1/4 cup feta cheese, crumbled
- 2 tbsp. olive oil
- 1 lemon (zest and juice)
- Fresh parsley for garnish

Instructions:

1. In a bowl, combine quinoa, tuna, tomatoes, cucumber, olives, feta, olive oil, lemon zest, and lemon juice.
2. Toss well and garnish with fresh parsley.

LIME BASIL SHRIMP SKEWERS

Preparation Time: 20 minutes (plus marinating time) Servings: 4

Nutrition per Serving: Calories: 210 Carbohydrates: 8g Protein: 24g Fat: 10g

Ingredients:

- 1 lb shrimp, peeled and deveined
- 2 limes (zest and juice)
- 2 tbsp. fresh basil, chopped
- 1 tbsp. olive oil
- 1 tsp honey
- Wooden skewers (presoaked)

Instructions:

1. In a bowl, mix lime zest, lime juice, basil, olive oil, and honey.
2. Marinate shrimp in the mixture for at least 30 minutes.
3. Thread shrimp onto skewers and grill in the Instant Pot on the sauté mode for 23 minutes per side.

SOY GINGER GLAZED SALMON

Preparation Time: 20 minutes   Servings: 2

Nutrition per Serving: Calories: 270 Carbohydrates: 15g Protein: 28g Fat: 12g

Ingredients:

- 2 salmon fillets
- 2 tbsp. low sodium soy sauce
- 1 tbsp. honey
- 1 tbsp. fresh ginger, grated
- 1 tbsp. sesame oil
- 1 tsp sesame seeds
- Green onions for garnish

Instructions:

1. In a bowl, mix soy sauce, honey, ginger, and sesame oil.
2. Brush the mixture over salmon fillets, sprinkle with sesame seeds.
3. Place fillets in Instant Pot, set to high pressure for 3 minutes, then quick release. Garnish with green onions.

SHRIMP AND AVOCADO SALAD

Preparation Time: 15 minutes Servings: 2

Nutrition per Serving: Calories: 230 Carbohydrates: 12g Protein: 20g Fat: 14g

Ingredients:

- 1 lb. shrimp, peeled and deveined
- 1 avocado, diced
- 1 cup cherry tomatoes, halved
- 1/4 cup red onion, finely chopped
- 2 tbsp. fresh cilantro, chopped
- 2 tbsp. olive oil
- 1 lime (zest and juice)
- Salt and pepper to taste

Instructions:

1. Set Instant Pot to sauté mode, sauté shrimp in olive oil.
2. In a bowl, combine shrimp, avocado, tomatoes, red onion, cilantro, lime zest, lime juice, salt, and pepper.
3. Toss gently and serve.

BEEF PORK AND LAMB RECIPES

BEEF AND VEGETABLE SOUP

Preparation Time: 15 minutes Servings: 6

Nutrition per Serving: Calories: 250, Carbs: 15g, Protein: 20g, Fat: 10g

Ingredients:

- 1 lb lean beef stew meat
- 1 onion, diced
- 2 carrots, sliced
- 2 celery stalks, chopped
- 1 can diced tomatoes
- 4 cups beef broth (low sodium)
- 1 tsp thyme
- Salt and pepper to taste

Instructions:

1. Sauté beef in Instant Pot, then add vegetables, tomatoes, broth, thyme, salt, and pepper.
2. Pressure cook on high for 20 minutes.

BALSAMIC GLAZED BEEF

Preparation Time: 15 minutes Servings: 4

Nutrition per Serving: Calories: 300, Carbs: 10g, Protein: 28g, Fat: 15g

Ingredients:

- 1.5 lbs beef sirloin, thinly sliced
- 1/4 cup balsamic vinegar
- 2 tbsp. olive oil
- 2 cloves garlic, minced
- 2 tbsp honey

Instructions:

1. Sauté beef in Instant Pot.
2. Mix balsamic vinegar, olive oil, honey, and garlic; pour over beef.
3. Pressure cook for 10 minutes.

BEEF AND CAULIFLOWER RICE STIR-FRY

Preparation Time: 20 minutes Servings: 4

Nutrition per Serving: Calories: 280, Carbs: 10g, Protein: 25g, Fat: 15g

Ingredients:

- 1 lb. lean beef strips
- 1 head cauliflower, riced
- 1 bell pepper, sliced
- 1 cup broccoli florets
- 2 tbsp. low sodium soy sauce
- 1 tbsp. sesame oil
- 2 cloves garlic, minced

Instructions:

1. Sauté beef in Instant Pot, then add cauliflower rice, bell pepper, broccoli, soy sauce, sesame oil, and garlic.
2. Pressure cook for 5 minutes.

PORK AND SWEET POTATO STEW

Preparation Time: 20 minutes Servings: 6

Nutrition per Serving: Calories: 280, Carbs: 20g, Protein: 18g, Fat: 12g

Ingredients:

- 1.5 lbs. pork loin, cubed
- 2 sweet potatoes, peeled and cubed
- 1 onion, diced
- 2 cloves garlic, minced
- 1 can diced tomatoes
- 4 cups low sodium chicken broth
- 1 tsp thyme
- Salt and pepper to taste

Instructions:

1. Sauté pork in Instant Pot.
2. Add sweet potatoes, onion, garlic, tomatoes, broth, thyme, salt, and pepper.
3. Pressure cook on high for 20 minutes.

PORK AND CABBAGE STIR-FRY

Preparation Time: 20 minutes Servings: 4

Nutrition per Serving: Calories: 250, Carbs: 15g, Protein: 22g, Fat: 12g

Ingredients:

- 1 lb. pork loin, thinly sliced
- 1/2 head cabbage, shredded
- 1 carrot, julienned
- 1/4 cup low sodium soy sauce
- 2 tbsp. rice vinegar
- 2 cloves garlic, minced
- 1 tbsp. sesame oil

Instructions:

1. Sauté pork in Instant Pot, then add cabbage, carrot, soy sauce, rice vinegar, sesame oil, and garlic.
2. Pressure cook for 6 minutes.

PULLED PORK LETTUCE WRAPS

Preparation Time: 15 minutes Servings: 6

Nutrition per Serving: Calories: 280, Carbs: 15g, Protein: 25g, Fat: 14g

Ingredients:

- 2 lbs. pork shoulder, shredded
- 1 cup barbecue sauce (sugar free)
- 1 tsp smoked paprika
- 1 tsp cumin
- Iceberg lettuce leaves for wrapping

Instructions:

1. Combine shredded pork, barbecue sauce, smoked paprika, and cumin in Instant Pot.
2. Pressure cook on high for 60 minutes.
3. Serve in lettuce wraps.

LAMB AND VEGETABLE STEW

Preparation Time: 15 minutes Servings: 4

Nutrition per Serving: Calories: 320, Carbs: 25g, Protein: 22g, Fat: 14g

Ingredients:

- 1 lb. lamb stew meat
- 1 onion, diced
- 2 carrots, sliced
- 1 cup green beans, chopped
- 1 can diced tomatoes
- 4 cups low sodium beef broth
- 1 tsp thyme
- Salt and pepper to taste

Instructions:

1. Sauté lamb in Instant Pot, then add vegetables, tomatoes, broth, thyme, salt, and pepper.
2. Pressure cook on high for 20 minutes.

MINTED LAMB CHOPS

Preparation Time: 15 minutes Servings: 4

Nutrition per Serving: Calories: 280, Carbs: 10g, Protein: 25g, Fat: 16g

Ingredients:

- 1.5 lbs lamb chops
- 1/4 cup fresh mint, chopped
- 2 tbsp. olive oil
- 2 cloves garlic, minced
- 1 tsp rosemary
- Salt and pepper to taste

Instructions:

1. Coat lamb chops with olive oil, mint, garlic, rosemary, salt, and pepper.
2. Sear in Instant Pot using sauté function.
3. Pressure cook for 12 minutes.

LAMB AND LENTIL STEW

Preparation Time: 20 minutes Servings: 6

Nutrition per Serving: Calories: 320, Carbs: 30g, Protein: 20g, Fat: 12g

Ingredients:

- 1.5 lbs. lamb shoulder, cubed
- 1 cup green lentils, rinsed
- 1 onion, diced
- 2 carrots, sliced
- 3 cups low sodium beef broth
- 2 tsp thyme
- Salt and pepper to taste

Instructions:

1. Sauté lamb in Instant Pot.
2. Add lentils, onion, carrots, broth, thyme, salt, and pepper.
3. Pressure cook on high for 20 minutes.

BEEF AND BROCCOLI QUINOA BOWL

Preparation Time: 20 minutes Servings: 4

Nutrition per Serving: Calories: 320, Carbs: 25g, Protein: 26g, Fat: 12g

Ingredients:

- 1 lb. lean beef strips
- 1 cup quinoa, cooked
- 2 cups broccoli florets
- 1 bell pepper, sliced
- 2 tbsp. low sodium soy sauce
- 1 tbsp. hoisin sauce
- 1 tsp sesame oil
- 2 cloves garlic, minced

Instructions:

1. Sauté beef in Instant Pot, then add broccoli, bell pepper, soy sauce, hoisin sauce, sesame oil, and garlic.
2. Serve over cooked quinoa.

BEEF AND BLACK BEAN CHILI

Preparation Time: 20 minutes Servings: 6

Nutrition per Serving: Calories: 280, Carbs: 20g, Protein: 25g, Fat: 12g

Ingredients:

- 1 lb lean ground beef
- 2 cans black beans (low sodium), drained
- 1 can diced tomatoes
- 1 onion, diced
- 2 cloves garlic, minced
- 2 tbsp chili powder
- 1 tsp cumin
- Salt and pepper to taste

Instructions:

1. Sauté ground beef in Instant Pot, then add onion and garlic.
2. Add black beans, diced tomatoes, chili powder, cumin, salt, and pepper.
3. Pressure cook for 15 minutes.

BEEF AND ZUCCHINI LASAGNA

Preparation Time: 25 minutes Servings: 6

Nutrition per Serving: Calories: 300, Carbs: 15g, Protein: 28g, Fat: 15g

Ingredients:

- 1 lb lean ground beef
- 2 zucchinis, thinly sliced
- 1 cup ricotta cheese (partskim)
- 1 cup marinara sauce (no added sugar)
- 1 cup mozzarella cheese, shredded
- 2 cloves garlic, minced
- 1 tsp Italian seasoning
- Salt and pepper to taste

Instructions:

1. Sauté ground beef in Instant Pot, then add garlic and marinara sauce.
2. In a separate bowl, mix ricotta cheese with Italian seasoning.
3. Layer zucchini slices, beef mixture, and ricotta in the Instant Pot. Repeat layers.
4. Top with mozzarella cheese.
5. Pressure cook for 15 minutes.

PORK AND VEGETABLE CURRY

Preparation Time: 25 minutes Servings: 4

Nutrition per Serving: Calories: 320, Carbs: 25g, Protein: 20g, Fat: 15g

Ingredients:

- 1.5 lbs pork loin, cubed
- 2 cups cauliflower florets
- 1 can chickpeas (low sodium), drained
- 1 onion, diced
- 2 tomatoes, chopped
- 2 tbsp curry powder
- 1 tsp cumin
- 1 tsp turmeric

Instructions:

1. Sauté pork in Instant Pot, then add cauliflower, chickpeas, onion, tomatoes, curry powder, cumin, and turmeric.
2. Pressure cook on high for 25 minutes.

PORK AND APPLE SKILLET

Preparation Time: 20 minutes Servings: 4

Nutrition per Serving: Calories: 290, Carbs: 20g, Protein: 22g, Fat: 14g

Ingredients:

- 1.5 lbs pork tenderloin, sliced
- 2 apples, sliced
- 1 onion, thinly sliced
- 1/4 cup apple cider vinegar
- 2 tbsp. honey
- 1 tsp cinnamon
- Salt and pepper to taste

Instructions:

1. Sauté pork in Instant Pot, then add apples, onion, apple cider vinegar, honey, cinnamon, salt, and pepper.
1. 2. Pressure cook for 10 minutes

PORK AND VEGETABLE KEBABS

Preparation Time: 15 minutes (plus margination time) Servings: 4

Nutrition per Serving: Calories: 280, Carbs: 15g, Protein: 24g, Fat: 14g

Ingredients:

- lbs. pork loin, cubed
- 1 zucchini, sliced
- 1 bell pepper, sliced
- 1 red onion, sliced
- 2 tbsp. olive oil
- 2 tbsp. balsamic vinegar
- 1 tsp dried oregano
- Salt and pepper to taste

Instructions:

1. Marinate pork in olive oil, balsamic vinegar, oregano, salt, and pepper for at least 1 hour.
2. Thread pork and vegetables onto skewers and cook in Instant Pot using the sauté function.

LAMB AND CHICKPEA TAGINE

Preparation Time: 25 minutes Servings: 4

Nutrition per Serving: Calories: 350, Carbs: 30g, Protein22g, Fat: 18g

Ingredients:

- 1 lb. lamb shoulder, cubed
- 1 can chickpeas (low sodium), drained
- 2 carrots, sliced
- 1 onion, diced
- 2 tomatoes, chopped
- 1/4 cup dried apricots, chopped
- 2 tbsp. olive oil
- 1 tsp ground cumin
- 1 tsp ground coriander

Instructions:

1. Sauté lamb in Instant Pot, then add chickpeas, carrots, onion, tomatoes, apricots, olive oil, cumin, and coriander.
2. Pressure cook on high for 20 minutes.

LAMB AND QUINOA STUFFED PEPPERS

Preparation Time: 25 minutes Servings: 4

Nutrition per Serving: Calories: 320, Carbs: 25g, Protein: 22g, Fat: 14g

Ingredients:

- 1 lb. ground lamb
- 1 cup quinoa, cooked
- 4 bell peppers, halved
- 1 can diced tomatoes
- 1 onion, diced
- 2 cloves garlic, minced
- 1 tsp cinnamon
- 1 tsp cumin
- Salt and pepper to taste

Instructions:

1. Sauté ground lamb in Instant Pot, then add onion, garlic, diced tomatoes, cinnamon, cumin, salt, and pepper.
2. Mix in cooked quinoa.
3. Stuff bell peppers with the lamb and quinoa mixture.
4. Pressure cook for 15 minutes.

LAMB AND CAULIFLOWER RICE PILAF

Preparation Time: 20 minutes Servings: 4

Nutrition per Serving: Calories: 330, Carbs: 20g, Protein: 26g, Fat: 16g

Ingredients:

- 1 lb lamb stew meat
- 1 head cauliflower, riced
- 1 cup peas
- 1 onion, diced
- 2 cloves garlic, minced
- 1 tsp cumin
- 1 tsp coriander
- 1/4 cup fresh cilantro, chopped

Instructions:

1. Sauté lamb in Instant Pot, then add cauliflower rice, peas, onion, garlic, cumin, and coriander.
2. Pressure cook for 8 minutes.
3. Garnish with fresh cilantro.

BEEF AND SPINACH STUFFED MUSHROOMS

Preparation Time: 20 minutes Servings: 4

Nutrition per Serving: Calories: 260, Carbs: 10g, Protein: 24g, Fat: 14g

Ingredients:

- 1 lb lean ground beef
- 1 cup spinach, chopped
- 1/2 cup feta cheese, crumbled
- 1/4 cup onion, finely chopped
- 1 clove garlic, minced
- 1 tsp Italian seasoning
- Salt and pepper to taste
- 12 large mushrooms, cleaned and stems removed

Instructions:

1. Sauté ground beef in Instant Pot, then add spinach, feta cheese, onion, garlic, Italian seasoning, salt, and pepper.
2. Stuff mushrooms with the beef mixture.
3. Pressure cook for 10 minutes.

PORK AND BEAN CASSEROLE

Preparation Time: 20 minutes Servings: 6

Nutrition per Serving: Calories: 290, Carbs: 25g, Protein: 22g, Fat: 14g

Ingredients:

- 1.5 lbs pork loin, cubed
- 2 cans cannellini beans (lowsodium), drained
- 1 cup cherry tomatoes, halved
- 1 onion, dice
- 2 cloves garlic, minced
- 1/4 cup fresh parsley, chopped
- 2 tbsp. olive oil
- 1 tsp smoked paprika
- Salt and pepper to taste

Instructions:

1. Sauté pork in Instant Pot, then add beans, tomatoes, onion, garlic, parsley, olive oil, smoked paprika, salt, and pepper.
2. Pressure cook on high for 20 minutes.

BEEF AND CABBAGE ROLL CASSEROLE

Preparation Time: 25 minutes Servings: 6

Nutrition per Serving: Calories: 280, Carbs: 20g, Protein: 25g, Fat: 12g

Ingredients:

- 1 lb. lean ground beef
- 1 head cabbage, shredded
- 1 cup rice, cooked
- 1 can tomato sauce (no added sugar)
- 1 onion, diced
- 2 cloves garlic, minced
- 1 tsp paprika
- Salt and pepper to taste

Instructions:

1. Sauté ground beef in Instant Pot, then add onion, garlic, tomato sauce, paprika, salt, and pepper.
2. Layer shredded cabbage and cooked rice over the beef mixture.
3. Pressure cook for 15 minutes.

PORK AND BUTTERNUT SQUASH STEW

Preparation Time: 25 minutes Servings: 4

Nutrition per Serving: Calories: 320, Carbs: 30g, Protein: 20g, Fat: 15g

Ingredients:

1.5 lbs. pork shoulder, cubed

1 butternut squash, peeled and diced

2 apples, peeled and sliced

1 onion, diced

4 cups low sodium chicken broth

2 tsp sage

1 tsp cinnamon

Salt and pepper to taste

Instructions:

1. Sauté pork in Instant Pot, then add butternut squash, apples, onion, broth, sage, cinnamon, salt, and pepper.

2. Pressure cook on high for 25 minutes

LAMB AND EGGPLANT CURRY

Preparation Time: 25 minutes Servings: 4

Nutrition per Serving: Calories: 350, Carbs: 30g, Protein: 22g, Fat: 18g

Ingredients:

- 1 lb lamb stew meat
- 1 large eggplant, diced
- 1 can chickpeas (low sodium), drained
- 1 onion, diced
- 2 tomatoes, chopped
- 2 tbsp curry powder
- 1 tsp cumin
- 1 tsp coriander

Instructions:

1. Sauté lamb in Instant Pot, then add eggplant, chickpeas, onion, tomatoes, curry powder, cumin, and coriander.

2. Pressure cook on high for 25 minutes

LAMB AND MUSHROOM RISOTTO

Preparation Time: 20 minutes Servings: 4

Nutrition per Serving: Calories: 330, Carbs: 25g, Protein: 26g, Fat: 16g

Ingredients:

1 lb. lamb sirloin, thinly sliced

1.5 cups Arborio rice

1 cup mushrooms, sliced

1 onion, finely chopped

4 cups beef broth (low sodium)

1/2 cup dry white wine

2 tbsp olive oil

2 cloves garlic, minced

Instructions:

1. Sauté lamb in Instant Pot, then add mushrooms, onion, garlic, rice, broth, and white wine.

2. Pressure cook on high for 7 minutes.

Preparation Time: 25 minutes Servings: 4

Nutrition per Serving: Calories: 320, Carbs: 25g, Protein: 22g, Fat: 14g

Ingredients:

- 1 lb. lamb stew meat
- 1 cup wild rice, cooked
- 1 cup asparagus, chopped
- 1/2 cup dried cranberries
- 1 onion, diced
- 2 cloves garlic, minced
- 4 cups low sodium chicken broth
- 2 tbsp. olive oil

Instructions:

1. Sauté lamb in Instant Pot, then add asparagus, onion, garlic, dried cranberries, rice, and chicken broth.
2. Pressure cook for 15 minutes.

VEGETABLES AND SIDE

GARLIC LEMON BROCCOLI

Preparation Time: 10 minutes Servings: 4

Nutrition per Serving: Calories: 50, Carbs: 8g, Protein: 3g, Fat: 2g

Ingredients:

- 4 cups broccoli florets
- 2 tbsp olive oil
- 3 cloves garlic, minced
- 1 lemon (zested and juiced)
- Salt and pepper to taste

Instructions:

1. Place broccoli in Instant Pot with olive oil, garlic, lemon zest, and juice.
2. Pressure cook on high for 2 minutes.

SESAME GINGER GREEN BEANS

Preparation Time: 12 minutes Servings: 4

Nutrition per Serving: Calories: 45, Carbs: 8g, Protein: 2g, Fat: 2g

Ingredients:

- 1 lb. green beans, trimmed
- 2 tbsp. soy sauce (low sodium)
- 1 tbsp. sesame oil
- 1 tbsp. rice vinegar
- 1 tsp fresh ginger, grated
- 1 tsp sesame seeds

Instructions:

1. Place green beans in Instant Pot with soy sauce, sesame oil, rice vinegar, ginger, and sesame seeds.
2. Pressure cook for 2 minutes.

SPICY CAULIFLOWER RICE

Preparation Time: 15 minutes Servings: 4

Nutrition per Serving: Calories: 60, Carbs: 10g, Protein: 3g, Fat: 2g

Ingredients:

- 1 head cauliflower, riced
- 1 tbsp. olive oil
- 1 tsp cumin
- 1/2 tsp chili powder
- 1/4 tsp cayenne pepper
- Salt and pepper to taste

Instructions:

1. Sauté cauliflower rice in Instant Pot with olive oil, cumin, chili powder, cayenne, salt, and pepper.
2. Pressure cook for 3 minutes.

MASHED GARLIC CAULIFLOWER

Preparation Time: 15 minutes Servings: 4

Nutrition per Serving: Calories: 70, Carbs: 8g, Protein: 3g, Fat: 4g

Ingredients:

- 1 head cauliflower, chopped
- 3 cloves garlic, minced
- 2 tbsp. butter (unsalted)
- 1/4 cup unsweetened almond milk
- Salt and pepper to taste

Instructions:

1. Steam cauliflower in Instant Pot until tender.
2. Mash cauliflower with garlic, butter, almond milk, salt, and pepper.
3. Serve warm.

. QUINOA PILAF WITH MIXED VEGETABLES

Preparation Time: 15 minutes Servings: 4

Nutrition per Serving: Calories: 180, Carbs: 30g, Protein: 6g, Fat: 4g

Ingredients:

- 1 cup quinoa, rinsed
- 2 cups mixed vegetables (peas, carrots, corn)
- 1 onion, finely chopped
- 2 cloves garlic, minced
- 2 cups vegetable broth (low sodium)
- 1 tbsp. olive oil
- Salt and pepper to taste

Instructions:

1. Sauté onion and garlic in Instant Pot with olive oil.
2. Add quinoa, mixed vegetables, vegetable broth, salt, and pepper.
3. Pressure cook for 5 minutes.

HERBED CARROT COINS

Preparation Time: 10 minutes Servings: 4

Nutrition per Serving: Calories: 60, Carbs: 14g, Protein: 1g, Fat: 1g

Ingredients:

- 4 large carrots, sliced
- 2 tbsp. olive oil
- 1 tsp dried thyme
- 1 tsp dried rosemary
- Salt and pepper to taste

Instructions:

1. Place carrot slices in Instant Pot with olive oil, thyme, rosemary, salt, and pepper.
2. Pressure cook for 4 minutes.

CILANTRO LIME BROWN RICE

Preparation Time: 12 minutes Servings: 4

Nutrition per Serving: Calories: 160, Carbs: 32g, Protein: 3g, Fat: 2g

Ingredients:

- 1 cup brown rice, rinsed
- 2 cups water
- 1/4 cup fresh cilantro, chopped
- 1 lime (zested and juiced)
- Salt to taste

Instructions:

1. Combine brown rice, water, cilantro, lime zest, and lime juice in Instant Pot.
2. Pressure cook for 7 minutes.

LEMON DILL ROASTED POTATOES

Preparation Time: 20 minutes Servings: 4

Nutrition per Serving: Calories: 140, Carbs: 30g, Protein: 3g, Fat: 1g

Ingredients:

- 1 lb. baby potatoes, halved
- 2 tbsp. olive oil
- 1 lemon (zested and juiced)
- 2 tbsp. fresh dill, chopped
- Salt and pepper to taste

Instructions:

1. Toss potatoes in Instant Pot with olive oil, lemon zest, lemon juice, dill, salt, and pepper.
2. Pressure cook for 5 minutes.

ROASTED BRUSSELS SPROUTS

Preparation Time: 15 minutes Servings: 4

Nutrition per Serving: Calories: 70, Carbs: 10g, Protein: 4g, Fat: 3g

Ingredients:

- 1 lb. Brussels sprouts, halved
- 2 tbsp. olive oil
- 1 tsp garlic powder
- Salt and pepper to taste

Instructions:

1. Toss Brussels sprouts in Instant Pot with olive oil, garlic powder, salt, and pepper.
2. Pressure cook for 3 minutes.
3. Broil in the oven for a crisp finish.

GARLIC HERB QUINOA

Preparation Time: 15 minutes Servings: 4

Nutrition per Serving: Calories: 160, Carbs: 30g, Protein: 5g, Fat: 2g

Ingredients:

- 1 cup quinoa, rinsed
- 2 cups vegetable broth (low sodium)
- 2 cloves garlic, minced
- 1 tsp dried thyme
- 1 tsp dried rosemary
- Salt and pepper to taste

Instructions:

1. Combine quinoa, vegetable broth, garlic, thyme, rosemary, salt, and pepper in Instant Pot.
2. Pressure cook for 5 minutes.

TURMERIC INFUSED CAULIFLOWER

Preparation Time: 12 minutes Servings: 4

Nutrition per Serving: Calories: 50, Carbs: 10g, Protein: 3g, Fat: 2g

Ingredients:

- 1 head cauliflower, chopped
- 1 tsp turmeric powder
- 1 tbsp olive oil
- 1/2 tsp cumin
- 1/2 tsp coriander
- Salt and pepper to taste

Instructions:

1. Sauté cauliflower in Instant Pot with turmeric powder, olive oil, cumin, coriander, salt, and pepper.
2. Pressure cook for 3 minutes

GARLIC PARMESAN ASPARAGUS

Preparation Time: 10 minutes Servings: 4

Nutrition per Serving: Calories: 60, Carbs: 5g, Protein: 4g, Fat: 4g

Ingredients:

- 1 lb. asparagus, trimmed
- 2 tbsp. grated Parmesan cheese
- 2 cloves garlic, minced
- 1 tbsp. olive oil
- Salt and pepper to taste

Instructions:

1. Toss asparagus in Instant Pot with Parmesan cheese, garlic, olive oil, salt, and pepper.
2. Pressure cook for 2 minutes.

BALSAMIC GLAZED BRUSSELS SPROUTS

Preparation Time: 15 minutes   Servings: 4

Nutrition per Serving: Calories: 80, Carbs: 15g, Protein: 4g, Fat: 3g

Ingredients:

- 1 lb. Brussels sprouts, halved
- 2 tbsp. balsamic vinegar
- 1 tbsp. olive oil
- 1 tsp honey
- Salt and pepper to taste

Instructions:

1. Toss Brussels sprouts in Instant Pot with balsamic vinegar, olive oil, honey, salt, and pepper.
2. Pressure cook for 3 minutes.

BUTTERNUT SQUASH RISOTTO

Preparation Time: 20 minutes Servings: 4

Nutrition per Serving: Calories: 220, Carbs: 45g, Protein: 5g, Fat: 3g

Ingredients:

1 cup Arborio rice

2 cups butternut squash, diced

1 onion, finely chopped

2 cloves garlic, minced

4 cups vegetable broth (low sodium)

2 tbsp. olive oil

Salt and pepper to taste

Instructions:

1. Sauté onion and garlic in Instant Pot with olive oil.
2. Add Arborio rice, butternut squash, vegetable broth, salt, and pepper.
3. Pressure cook for 7 minutes.

SAUTÉED LEMON GARLIC SPINACH

Preparation Time: 8 minutes Servings: 4

Nutrition per Serving: Calories: 40, Carbs: 5g, Protein: 3g, Fat: 2g

Ingredients:

- 1 lb fresh spinach
- 2 cloves garlic, minced
- 1 lemon (zested and juiced)
- 1 tbsp olive oil
- Salt and pepper to taste

Instructions:

1. Sauté spinach in Instant Pot with olive oil, garlic, lemon zest, and juice.
2. Pressure cook for 1 minute

CUMIN INFUSED LENTILS

Preparation Time: 15 minutes Servings: 4

Nutrition per Serving: Calories: 160, Carbs: 25g, Protein: 9g, Fat: 2g

Ingredients:

- 1 cup dried green lentils, rinsed
- 3 cups water
- 1 onion, finely chopped
- 2 cloves garlic, minced
- 1 tsp cumin
- 1 tsp coriander
- 1 tbsp. olive oil
- Salt and pepper to taste

Instructions:

1. Sauté onion and garlic in Instant Pot with olive oil.
2. Add lentils, water, cumin, coriander, salt, and pepper.
3. Pressure cook for 8 minutes.

BALSAMIC GLAZED CARROTS

Preparation Time: 12 minutes Servings: 4

Nutrition per Serving: Calories: 80, Carbs: 18g, Protein: 1g, Fat: 1g

Ingredients:

- 1 lb. baby carrots
- 2 tbsp. balsamic vinegar
- 1 tbsp. olive oil
- 1 tbsp. honey
- Salt and pepper to taste

Instructions:

1. Toss carrots in Instant Pot with balsamic vinegar, olive oil, honey, salt, and pepper.
2. Pressure cook for 3 minutes.

ROSEMARY INFUSED SWEET POTATOES

Preparation Time: 15 minutes Servings: 4

Nutrition per Serving: Calories: 120, Carbs: 28g, Protein: 2g, Fat: 1g

Ingredients:

- 2 large sweet potatoes, peeled and diced
- 2 tbsp. olive oil
- 1 tsp dried rosemary
- Salt and pepper to taste

Instructions:

1. Toss sweet potatoes in Instant Pot with olive oil, dried rosemary, salt, and pepper.
2. Pressure cook for 5 minutes.

LEMON HERB QUINOA SALAD

Preparation Time: 15 minutes Servings: 4

Nutrition per Serving: Calories: 180, Carbs: 30g, Protein: 5g, Fat: 5g

Ingredients:

- 1 cup quinoa, cooked
- 1 cup cherry tomatoes, halved
- 1 cucumber, diced
- 1/4 cup fresh parsley, chopped
- 1/4 cup feta cheese, crumbled
- 1 lemon (zested and juiced)
- 2 tbsp. olive oil
- Salt and pepper to taste

Instructions:

1. Combine quinoa, tomatoes, cucumber, parsley, feta cheese, lemon zest, lemon juice, olive oil, salt, and pepper in Instant Pot.
2. Mix well.

Instructions:

HONEY GLAZED BUTTERNUT SQUASH

Preparation Time: 12 minutes Servings: 4

Nutrition per Serving: Calories: 120, Carbs: 30g, Protein: 2g, Fat: 1g

Ingredients:

- 4 cups butternut squash, diced
- 2 tbsp honey
- 1 tbsp olive oil
- 1 tsp cinnamon
- Salt and pepper to taste

Instructions:

1. Toss butternut squash in Instant Pot with honey, olive oil, cinnamon, salt, and pepper.
2. Pressure cook for 4 minutes.

MUSHROOM AND THYME RISOTTO

Preparation Time: 20 minutes Servings: 4

Nutrition per Serving: Calories: 220, Carbs: 45g, Protein: 5g, Fat: 2g

Ingredients:

- 1 cup Arborio rice
- 2 cups mushrooms, sliced
- 1 onion, finely chopped
- 2 cloves garlic, minced
- 4 cups vegetable broth (lowsodium)
- 2 tbsp fresh thyme, chopped
- 2 tbsp olive oil
- Salt and pepper to taste

1. Sauté onion and garlic in Instant Pot with olive oil.
2. Add Arborio rice, mushrooms, vegetable broth, thyme, salt, and pepper.
3. Pressure cook for 7 minutes.

CUMIN LIME BLACK BEANS

Preparation Time: 15 minutes Servings: 4

Nutrition per Serving: Calories: 160, Carbs: 27g, Protein: 7g, Fat: 2g

Ingredients:

- 2 cans black beans (low sodium), drained
- 1 onion, finely chopped
- 2 cloves garlic, minced
- 1 tsp cumin
- 1 lime (zested and juiced)
- 2 tbsp. fresh cilantro, chopped
- 1 tbsp. olive oil
- Salt and pepper to taste

Instructions:

1. Sauté onion and garlic in Instant Pot with olive oil.
2. Add black beans, cumin, lime zest, lime juice, cilantro, salt, and pepper.
3. Pressure cook for 5 minutes.

2   Pressure cook for 2 minutes.

CRISPY GARLIC PARMESAN BRUSSELS SPROUTS

Preparation Time: 15 minutes Servings: 4

Nutrition per Serving: Calories: 120, Carbs: 12g, Protein: 5g, Fat: 7g

Ingredients:

- 1 lb. Brussels sprouts, halved
- 2 tbsp. olive oil
- 1/4 cup grated Parmesan cheese
- 3 cloves garlic, minced
- Salt and pepper to taste

Instructions:

1. Toss Brussels sprouts in Instant Pot with olive oil, Parmesan cheese, garlic, salt, and pepper.
2. Pressure cook for 4 minutes.

SAUTÉED GARLIC PARMESAN ZUCCHINI

Preparation Time: 10 minutes Servings: 4

Nutrition per Serving: Calories: 70, Carbs: 6g, Protein: 3g, Fat: 5g

Ingredients:

- 4 zucchinis, sliced
- 2 tbsp grated Parmesan cheese
- 2 cloves garlic, minced
- 2 tbsp olive oil
- Salt and pepper to taste

Instructions:

1. Sauté zucchini in Instant Pot with olive oil, Parmesan cheese, garlic, salt, and pepper

TURMERIC INFUSED QUINOA SALAD

Preparation Time: 15 minutes Servings: 4

Nutrition per Serving: Calories: 180, Carbs: 30g, Protein: 5g, Fat: 4g

Ingredients:

- 1 cup quinoa, cooked
- 1 cup cucumber, diced
- 1 cup cherry tomatoes, halved
- 1/4 cup red onion, finely chopped
- 2 tbsp olive oil
- 1 tsp turmeric powder
- 1 lemon (zested and juiced)
- Salt and pepper to taste

Instructions:

1. Combine quinoa, cucumber, tomatoes, red onion, olive oil, turmeric powder, lemon zest, lemon juice, salt, and pepper in Instant Pot.
2. Mix well.

LENTIL AND VEGETABLE SOUP

Preparation Time: 20 minutes Servings: 6

Nutrition per Serving: Calories: 200, Carbs: 30g, Protein: 12g, Fat: 3g

Ingredients:

- 1 cup lentils, rinsed
- 1 onion, diced
- 2 carrots, sliced
- 2 celery stalks, chopped
- 1 can diced tomatoes
- 4 cups vegetable broth (low sodium)
- 2 cloves garlic, minced
- 1 tsp cumin
- Salt and pepper to taste

Instructions:

1. Combine lentils, vegetables, tomatoes, broth, garlic, cumin, salt, and pepper in Instant Pot.
2. Pressure cook on high for 15 minutes.

CHICKPEA AND SPINACH CURRY

Preparation Time: 25 minutes Servings: 4

Nutrition per Serving: Calories: 280, Carbs: 40g, Protein: 14g, Fat: 8g

Ingredients:

- 2 cans chickpeas (low sodium), drained
- 1 onion, diced
- 2 tomatoes, chopped
- 2 cups spinach
- 1 can coconut milk (light)
- 2 tbsp. curry powder
- 1 tsp turmeric
- Salt and pepper to taste

Instructions:

2 Sauté onion in Instant Pot, then add chickpeas, tomatoes, spinach, coconut milk, curry powder, turmeric, salt, and pepper.
3 Pressure cook on high for 10 minutes.

QUINOA AND BLACK BEAN STUFFED BELL PEPPERS

Preparation Time: 25 minutes Servings: 4

Nutrition per Serving: Calories: 320, Carbs: 45g, Protein: 15g, Fat: 8g

Ingredients:

- 1 cup quinoa, cooked
- 1 can black beans (low sodium), drained
- 4 bell peppers, halved
- 1 cup corn kernels
- 1 cup salsa (no added sugar)
- 1 cup shredded vegan cheese
- 1 tsp cumin
- 1 tsp chili powder

Instructions:

1. Mix quinoa, black beans, corn, salsa, cumin, and chili powder in a bowl.
2. Stuff bell peppers with the mixture and top with vegan cheese.
3. Pressure cook for 15 minutes.

SWEET POTATO AND LENTIL CURRY

Preparation Time: 25 minutes Servings: 4

Nutrition per Serving: Calories: 300, Carbs: 40g, Protein: 15g, Fat: 8g

Ingredients:

- 1 cup red lentils, rinsed
- 2 sweet potatoes, peeled and diced
- 1 can coconut milk (light)
- 1 onion, diced
- 2 tbsp. curry powder
- 1 tsp ginger, grated
- 2 tomatoes, chopped
- Salt and pepper to taste

Instructions:

2. Sauté onion in Instant Pot, then add lentils, sweet potatoes, coconut milk, tomatoes, curry powder, ginger, salt, and pepper.
3. Pressure cook on high for 15 minutes

SPINACH AND MUSHROOM RISOTTO

Preparation Time: 20 minutes   Servings: 4

Nutrition per Serving: Calories: 280, Carbs: 35g, Protein: 10g, Fat: 10g

Ingredients:

- cups Arborio rice
- 1 onion, finely chopped
- 2 cups mushrooms, sliced
- 4 cups vegetable broth (low sodium)
- 2 cups fresh spinach
- 1/2 cup dry white wine
- 2 tbsp. olive oil
- 2 cloves garlic, minced

Instructions:

2. Sauté onion and mushrooms in Instant Pot, then add rice, broth, spinach, wine, olive oil, and garlic.
3. Pressure cook on high for 7 minutes.

CAULIFLOWER AND CHICKPEA CURRY

Preparation Time: 20 minutes Servings: 4

Nutrition per Serving: Calories: 250, Carbs: 30g, Protein: 12g, Fat: 10g

Ingredients:

- 1 head cauliflower, cut into florets
- 1 can chickpeas (low sodium), drained
- 1 onion, diced
- 2 tomatoes, chopped
- 1 can coconut milk (light)
- 2 tbsp curry powder
- 1 tsp turmeric
- 2 tbsp olive oil
- Salt and pepper to taste

Instructions:

1. Sauté onion in Instant Pot, then add cauliflower, chickpeas, tomatoes, coconut milk, curry powder, turmeric, olive oil, salt, and pepper.
2. Pressure cook on high for 10 minutes.

BUTTERNUT SQUASH AND SAGE RISOTTO

Preparation Time: 25 minutes Servings: 4

Nutrition per Serving: Calories: 300, Carbs: 40g, Protein: 8g, Fat: 10g

Ingredients:

- cups Arborio rice
- 1 butternut squash, peeled and diced
- 1 onion, finely chopped
- 4 cups vegetable broth (low sodium)
- 2 tbsp. olive oil
- 2 tbsp. fresh sage, chopped
- Salt and pepper to taste

Instructions:

2. Sauté onion in Instant Pot, then add rice, butternut squash, broth, sage, olive oil, salt, and pepper.
3. Pressure cook on high for 7 minutes.

EGGPLANT AND TOMATO STEW

Preparation Time: 20 minutes Servings: 4

Nutrition per Serving: Calories: 220, Carbs: 25g, Protein: 8g, Fat: 10g

Ingredients:

- 2 eggplants, diced
- 4 tomatoes, chopped
- 1 onion, finely chopped
- 2 cloves garlic, minced
- 2 tbsp. olive oil
- 1 tsp dried oregano
- 1 tsp basil
- Salt and pepper to taste

Instructions:

2. Sauté onion and garlic in Instant Pot, then add eggplant, tomatoes, olive oil, oregano, basil, salt, and pepper.
3. Pressure cook on high for 8 minutes.

BROCCOLI AND POTATO SOUP

Preparation Time: 20 minutes Servings: 6

Nutrition per Serving: Calories: 180, Carbs: 30g, Protein: 8g, Fat: 5g

Ingredients:

- 2 cups broccoli florets
- 4 potatoes, peeled and diced
- 1 onion, diced
- 2 cloves garlic, minced
- 4 cups vegetable broth (low sodium)
- 1 cup almond milk (unsweetened)
- 2 tbsp. nutritional yeast
- Salt and pepper to taste

Instructions:

1. Sauté onion and garlic in Instant Pot, then add broccoli, potatoes, broth, almond milk, nutritional yeast, salt, and pepper.
2. Pressure cook on high for 10 minutes.

CAULIFLOWER AND BROCCOLI GRATIN

Preparation Time: 25 minutes Servings: 6

Nutrition per Serving: Calories: 250, Carbs: 20g, Protein: 12g, Fat: 14g

Ingredients:

- 1 head cauliflower, cut into florets
- 2 cups broccoli florets
- 2 cups almond milk (unsweetened)
- 1/2 cup nutritional yeast
- 2 tbsp whole wheat flour
- 1 tsp Dijon mustard
- 2 tbsp olive oil
- Salt and pepper to taste

Instructions:

2. Sauté cauliflower and broccoli in Instant Pot, then add almond milk, nutritional yeast, flour, olive oil, mustard, salt, and pepper.
3. Pressure cook on high for 10 minutes.

SPAGHETTI SQUASH PRIMAVERA

Preparation Time: 20 minutes Servings: 4

Nutrition per Serving: Calories: 220, Carbs: 30g, Protein: 6g, Fat: 10g

Ingredients:

- 1 spaghetti squash, halved and seeded
- 2 cups cherry tomatoes, halved
- 1 zucchini, sliced
- 1 bell pepper, sliced
- 2 cloves garlic, minced
- 2 tbsp. olive oil
- 1 tsp dried basil
- 1 tsp dried oregano
- Salt and pepper to taste

Instructions:

2. Place spaghetti squash halves in Instant Pot, add vegetables, garlic, olive oil, basil, oregano, salt, and pepper.
3. Pressure cook on high for 10 minutes.

ZUCCHINI NOODLES WITH PESTO

Preparation Time: 15 minutes Servings: 4

Nutrition per Serving: Calories: 180, Carbs: 10g, Protein: 5g, Fat: 15g

Ingredients:

- 4 zucchinis, spiralizer
- 1 cup cherry tomatoes, halved
- 1/2 cup pine nuts
- 1 cup fresh basil leaves
- 2 cloves garlic
- 1/2 cup olive oil
- 1/2 cup grated Parmesan cheese
- Salt and pepper to taste

Instructions:

1. Sauté zucchini in Instant Pot, then add tomatoes.
2. In a blender, combine pine nuts, basil, garlic, olive oil, Parmesan, salt, and pepper to make pesto.
3. Mix zucchini with pesto.

RATATOUILLE

Preparation Time: 25 minutes Servings: 6

Nutrition per Serving: Calories: 180, Carbs: 25g, Protein: 5g, Fat: 8g

Ingredients:

- 2 zucchinis, sliced
- 1 eggplant, diced
- 1 bell pepper, sliced
- 2 tomatoes, sliced
- 1 onion, sliced
- 2 cloves garlic, minced
- 2 tbsp. olive oil
- 2 tomatoes, chopped
- 1 tsp dried thyme
- 1 tsp dried rosemary
- Salt and pepper to taste

Instructions:

2 Sauté onion and garlic in Instant Pot, then add zucchinis, eggplant, bell pepper, tomatoes, olive oil, thyme, rosemary, salt, and pepper.

3 Pressure cook on high for 10 minutes

STUFFED PORTOBELLO MUSHROOMS

Preparation Time: 20 minutes Servings: 4

Nutrition per Serving: Calories: 240, Carbs: 15g, Protein: 12g, Fat: 15g

Ingredients:

- 4 large Portobello mushrooms, stems removed
- 1 cup quinoa, cooked
- 1 cup spinach, chopped
- 1/2 cup feta cheese, crumbled
- 1/4 cup sun dried tomatoes, chopped
- 2 cloves garlic, minced
- 2 tbsp. olive oil
- Salt and pepper to taste

Instructions:

- Sauté mushrooms in Instant Pot, then mix quinoa, spinach, feta, tomatoes, garlic, olive oil, salt, and pepper.
- 2. Stuff mushrooms with the mixture and pressure cook for 10 minutes

BLACK BEAN AND QUINOA STUFFED PEPPERS

Preparation Time: 25 minutes Servings: 4

Nutrition per Serving: Calories: 280, Carbs: 40g, Protein: 15g, Fat: 8g

Ingredients:

- 1 cup quinoa, cooked
- 1 can black beans (low sodium), drained
- 4 bell peppers, halved
- 1 cup corn kernels
- 1 cup salsa (no added sugar)
- 1 cup shredded vegan cheese
- 1 tsp cumin
- 1 tsp chili powder

Instructions:

1. Mix quinoa, black beans, corn, salsa, vegan cheese, cumin, and chili powder in a bowl.
2. Stuff bell peppers with the mixture and pressure cook for 15 minutes.

PUMPKIN AND CHICKPEA CURRY

Preparation Time: 25 minutes Servings: 4

Nutrition per Serving: Calories: 270, Carbs: 35g, Protein: 12g, Fat: 10g

Ingredients:

- 1 can chickpeas (low sodium), drained
- 1 cup pumpkin puree
- 1 can coconut milk (light)
- 1 onion, diced
- 2 tbsp. curry powder
- 1 tsp ginger, grated
- Salt and pepper to taste

Instructions:

2 Sauté onion in Instant Pot, then add chickpeas, pumpkin puree, coconut milk, tomatoes, curry powder, ginger, salt, and pepper.
3 Pressure cook on high for 15 minutes

MUSHROOM AND SPINACH FRITTATA

Preparation Time: 20 minutes Servings: 4

Nutrition per Serving: Calories: 220, Carbs: 10g, Protein: 14g, Fat: 15g

Ingredients:

- 8 eggs
- 2 cups mushrooms, sliced
- 2 cups spinach
- 1 onion, diced
- 1/2 cup feta cheese, crumbled
- 2 tbsp. olive oil
- 1 tsp dried thyme
- Salt and pepper to taste

Instructions:

- Sauté mushrooms and onion in Instant Pot, then add spinach until wilted.
- Whisk eggs, feta, thyme, salt, and pepper in a bowl. Pour over the vegetables in the Instant Pot.
- Pressure cook on high for 8 minutes.

SPINACH AND ARTICHOKE RISOTTO

Preparation Time: 25 minutes Servings: 4

Nutrition per Serving: Calories: 290, Carbs: 35g, Protein: 10g, Fat: 12g

Ingredients:

- cups Arborio rice 1.5 (cups)
- 2 cups spinach
- 1 can artichoke hearts, chopped
- 4 cups vegetable broth (low sodium)
- 2 tbsp. nutritional yeast
- 2 tbsp. olive oil
- 2 cloves garlic, minced
- Salt and pepper to taste

Instructions:

1. Sauté garlic in Instant Pot, then add rice, spinach, artichokes, broth, nutritional yeast, olive oil, salt, and pepper.
2. Pressure cook on high for 7 minutes.

AVOCADO AND BLACK BEAN SALAD

Preparation Time: 15 minutes Servings: 4

Nutrition per Serving: Calories: 230, Carbs: 25g, Protein: 8g, Fat: 12g

Ingredients:

- 2 cans black beans (low sodium), drained
- 2 avocados, diced
- 1 cup cherry tomatoes, halved
- 1/2 cup red onion, finely chopped
- 2 tbsp. lime juice
- 1/4 cup nutritional yeast
- 1/4 cup cilantro, chopped
- 2 tbsp. olive oil
- Salt and pepper to taste

Instructions:

2. Mix black beans, avocados, tomatoes, onion, cilantro, lime juice, olive oil, salt, and pepper in a bowl.

SWEET POTATO AND CHICKPEA STEW

Preparation Time: 20 minutes   Servings: 4

Nutrition per Serving: Calories: 260, Carbs: 40g, Protein: 10g, Fat: 8g

Ingredients:

- 2 sweet potatoes, peeled and diced
- 1 can chickpeas (low sodium), drained
- 1 onion, diced
- 2 cups vegetable broth (low sodium)
- 2 tomatoes, chopped
- 2 tbsp. olive oil
- 1 tsp cumin
- 1 tsp paprika
- Salt and pepper to taste

Instructions:

2. Sauté onion in Instant Pot, then add sweet potatoes, chickpeas, broth, tomatoes, olive oil, cumin, paprika, salt, and pepper.
3. Pressure cook on high for 10 minutes.

QUINOA AND VEGETABLE STIRFRY

Preparation Time: 20 minutes Servings: 4

Nutrition per Serving: Calories: 250, Carbs: 35g, Protein: 10g, Fat: 8g

Ingredients:

- 1 cup quinoa, cooked
- 2 cups mixed vegetables (broccoli, bell peppers, snap peas)
- 1 cup tofu, cubed
- 2 tbsp. soy sauce (low sodium)
- 1 tbsp. sesame oil
- 1 tsp ginger, grated
- 2 cloves garlic, minced
- 1 tsp sesame seeds

Instructions:

1. Sauté tofu in Instant Pot, then add vegetables, quinoa, soy sauce, sesame oil, ginger, garlic, and sesame seeds.
2. Pressure cook on high for 5 minutes.

ARTICHOKE AND SPINACH STUFFED MUSHROOMS

Preparation Time: 20 minutes Servings: 4

Nutrition per Serving: Calories: 220, Carbs: 15g, Protein: 10g, Fat: 15g

Ingredients:

- 12 large mushrooms, cleaned and stems removed
- 2 cups spinach
- 1 can artichoke hearts, chopped
- 1 cup vegan cream cheese
- 2 cloves garlic, minced
- Salt and pepper to taste

Instructions:

2. Sauté spinach in Instant Pot, then mix with artichokes, vegan cream cheese, nutritional yeast, garlic, salt, and pepper.
3. Stuff mushrooms with the mixture and pressure cook for 10 minutes.

EGGPLANT AND LENTIL CASSEROLE

Preparation Time: 25 minutes Servings: 6

Nutrition per Serving: Calories: 260, Carbs: 35g, Protein: 12g, Fat: 8g

Ingredients:

- 2 eggplants, diced
- 1 cup lentils, rinsed
- 1 onion, diced
- 2 tomatoes, chopped
- 2 cups vegetable broth (low sodium)
- 2 tbsp. olive oil
- 1 tsp cumin
- 1 tsp paprika
- Salt and pepper to taste

Instructions:

2. Sauté onion in Instant Pot, then add eggplants, lentils, tomatoes, broth, olive oil, cumin, paprika, salt, and pepper.
3. Pressure cook on high for 15 minutes.

Preparation Time: 15 minutes Servings: 4

Nutrition per Serving: Calories: 220, Carbs: 30g, Protein: 8g, Fat: 8g

Ingredients:

- 1 cup quinoa, cooked
- 1 cucumber, diced
- 1 cup cherry tomatoes, halved
- 1/2 cup Kalamata olives, sliced
- 1/2 cup feta cheese, crumbled
- 1/4 cup red onion, finely chopped
- 2 tbsp. olive oil
- 2 tbsp. red wine vinegar
- 1 tsp dried oregano
- Salt and pepper to taste

Instructions:

1. Mix quinoa, cucumber, tomatoes, olives, feta, onion, olive oil, vinegar, oregano, salt, and pepper in a bowl.

CHICKPEA AND CAULIFLOWER CURRY

Preparation Time: 25 minutes Servings: 4

Nutrition per Serving: Calories: 290, Carbs: 40g, Protein: 14g, Fat: 10g

Ingredients:

- 1 can chickpeas (low sodium), drained
- 1 head cauliflower, cut into florets
- 1 onion, diced
- 2 tomatoes, chopped
- 1 can coconut milk (light)
- 2 tbsp. curry powder
- 1 tsp turmeric
- 2 tbsp. olive oil
- Salt and pepper to taste

Instructions:

- Sauté onion in Instant Pot, then add chickpeas, cauliflower, tomatoes, coconut milk, curry powder, turmeric, olive oil, salt, and pepper.
- Pressure cook on high for 10 minutes.

BEANS AND GRAINS

CHICKPEA AND SPINACH STEW

Preparation Time: 25 minutes Servings: 4

Nutrition per Serving: Calories: 250, Carbs: 35g, Protein: 14g, Fat: 7g

Ingredients:

- 2 cans chickpeas (low sodium), drained
- 1 onion, diced
- 2 tomatoes, chopped
- 3 cups fresh spinach
- 2 cloves garlic, minced
- 2 tsp cumin
- 1 tsp coriander
- 1/4 cup fresh cilantro, chopped

Instructions:

1. Sauté onion and garlic in Instant Pot.
2. Add chickpeas, tomatoes, spinach, cumin, coriander, and cilantro.
3. Pressure cook for 10 minutes.

BLACK BEAN SOUP

Preparation Time: 20 minutes Servings: 6

Nutrition per Serving: Calories: 220, Carbs: 30g, Protein: 12g, Fat: 5g

Ingredients:

- 2 cans black beans (low sodium), drained
- 1 onion, diced
- 2 carrots, sliced
- 2 stalks celery, chopped
- 4 cups vegetable broth (low sodium)
- 1 tsp cumin
- 1 tsp smoked paprika
- Salt and pepper to taste

Instructions:

1. Sauté onion, carrots, and celery in Instant Pot.
2. Add black beans, vegetable broth, cumin, smoked paprika, salt, and pepper.
3. . Pressure cook on high for 15 minutes

Preparation Time: 20 minutes Servings: 4

Nutrition per Serving: Calories: 280, Carbs: 35g, Protein: 15g, Fat: 8g

Ingredients:

- 1 cup red lentils, rinsed
- 1 can coconut milk (light)
- 1 onion, diced
- 2 tomatoes, chopped
- 2 tbsp curry powder
- 1 tsp turmeric
- 2 cloves garlic, minced

Instructions:

1. Sauté onion and garlic in Instant Pot.
2. Add red lentils, coconut milk, tomatoes, curry powder, turmeric, and a pinch of salt.
3. Pressure cook on high for 8 minutes.

PINTO BEAN AND QUINOA CHILI

Preparation Time: 20 minutes Servings: 6

Nutrition per Serving: Calories: 240, Carbs: 40g, Protein: 14g, Fat: 5g

Ingredients:

- 2 cups dried pinto beans, soaked overnight
- 1 cup quinoa, rinsed
- 1 can diced tomatoes
- 1 onion, diced
- 2 cloves garlic, minced
- 2 tbsps. chili powder
- 1 tsp cumin
- 4 cups vegetable broth (low sodium)

Instructions:

1. Sauté onion and garlic in Instant Pot.
2. Add soaked pinto beans, quinoa, diced tomatoes, chili powder, cumin, and enough water to cover.
3. Pressure cook on high for 20 minutes.

WHITE BEAN AND KALE STEW

Preparation Time: 25 minutes Servings: 6

Nutrition per Serving: Calories: 210, Carbs: 30g, Protein: 10g, Fat: 6g

Ingredients:

- 2 cans white beans (cannellini), drained
- 1 bunch kale, chopped
- 1 onion, diced
- 2 carrots, sliced
- 4 cups vegetable broth (lowsodium)
- 2 cloves garlic, minced
- 1 tsp thyme

Instructions:

1. Sauté onion, carrots, and garlic in Instant Pot.
2. Add white beans, kale, vegetable broth, thyme, salt, and pepper.
3. Pressure cook for 15 minutes.

BROWN RICE PILAF WITH VEGETABLES

Preparation Time: 25 minutes Servings: 4

Nutrition per Serving: Calories: 220, Carbs: 45g, Protein: 5g, Fat: 4g

Ingredients:

- 2 cups brown rice, rinsed
- 1 onion, diced
- 1 carrot, diced
- 1 zucchini, diced
- 4 cups vegetable broth (low sodium)
- 2 tbsp. olive oil
- 1 tsp thyme
- Salt and pepper to taste

Instructions:

1. Sauté onion in Instant Pot with olive oil.
2. Add brown rice, carrot, zucchini, vegetable broth, thyme, salt, and pepper.
3. Pressure cook for 15 minutes.

WILD RICE AND MUSHROOM PILAF

Preparation Time: 25 minutes Servings: 4

Nutrition per Serving: Calories: 230, Carbs: 40g, Protein: 8g, Fat: 5g

Ingredients:

- 1 cup wild rice, rinsed
- 1 cup mushrooms, sliced
- 1 onion, diced
- 2 cloves garlic, minced
- 2 tbsp. olive oil
- 1 tsp thyme
- Salt and pepper to taste

Instructions:

1. Sauté onion, garlic, and mushrooms in Instant Pot with olive oil.
2. Add wild rice, vegetable broth, thyme, salt, and pepper.
3. Pressure cook for 15 minutes

QUINOA SALAD WITH CHICKPEAS AND VEGGIES

Preparation Time: 15 minutes Servings: 4

Nutrition per Serving: Calories: 250, Carbs: 40g, Protein: 10g, Fat: 6g

Ingredients:

- 1 cup quinoa, cooked
- 1 can chickpeas (low sodium), drained
- 1 cucumber, diced
- 1 bell pepper, diced
- 1/4 cup feta cheese, crumbled
- 2 tbsp. olive oil
- 1 tbsp. balsamic vinegar
- 1 tsp Dijon mustard
- Salt and pepper to taste

Instructions:

1. Mix quinoa, chickpeas, cucumber, bell pepper, and feta in Instant Pot.
2. In a small bowl, whisk together olive oil, balsamic vinegar, mustard, salt, and pepper. Pour over the quinoa mixture.

MILLET AND BLACK BEAN STUFFED PEPPERS

Preparation Time: 20 minutes Servings: 4

Nutrition per Serving: Calories: 260, Carbs: 45g, Protein: 10g, Fat: 5g

Ingredients:

- 1 cup millet, cooked
- 1 can black beans (low sodium), drained
- 4 bell peppers, halved
- 1 cup corn kernels (fresh or frozen)
- 1 cup salsa (no added sugar)
- 1 tsp cumin
- 1/2 tsp chili powder

Instructions:

1. Mix cooked millet, black beans, corn, salsa, cumin, and chili powder in Instant Pot.
2. Stuff bell peppers with the mixture.
3. Pressure cook for 10 minutes.

THREE BEAN QUINOA SALAD

Preparation Time: 15 minutes Servings: 4

Nutrition per Serving: Calories: 230, Carbs: 40g, Protein: 10g, Fat: 5g

Ingredients:

- 1 cup quinoa, cooked
- 1 can black beans (low sodium), drained
- 1 can kidney beans (low sodium), drained
- 1 can chickpeas (low sodium), drained
- 1 bell pepper, diced
- 1/4 cup red onion, finely chopped
- 2 tbsp. olive oil
- 1 tbsp. red wine vinegar
- 1 tsp cumin
- Salt and pepper to taste

Instructions:

1. In a large bowl, combine quinoa, black beans, kidney beans, chickpeas, bell pepper, and red onion.
2. In a small bowl, whisk together olive oil, red wine vinegar, cumin, salt, and pepper. Pour over the quinoa mixture.

BARLEY AND VEGETABLE SOUP

Preparation Time: 25 minutes Servings: 6

Nutrition per Serving: Calories: 210, Carbs: 45g, Protein: 7g, Fat: 3g

Ingredients:

- 1 cup barley, rinsed
- 2 carrots, sliced
- 2 celery stalks, chopped
- 1 onion, diced
- 4 cups vegetable broth (low sodium)
- 2 tomatoes, chopped
- 1 tsp thyme
- Salt and pepper to taste

Instructions:

1. Sauté onion, carrots, and celery in Instant Pot.
2. Add barley, vegetable broth, tomatoes, thyme, salt, and pepper.

LENTIL AND BROWN RICE CASSEROLE

Preparation Time: 25 minutes Servings: 6

Nutrition per Serving: Calories: 220, Carbs: 40g, Protein: 10g, Fat: 4g

Ingredients:

- 1 cup brown rice, rinsed
- 1 cup green or brown lentils, rinsed
- 1 onion, diced
- 2 carrots, sliced
- 1 can diced tomatoes
- 4 cups vegetable broth (low sodium)
- 2 tsp Italian seasoning
- Salt and pepper to taste

Instructions:

1. Sauté onion in Instant Pot.
2. Add brown rice, lentils, diced tomatoes, vegetable broth, Italian seasoning, salt, and pepper.
3. Pressure cook on high for 20 minutes.

MEDITERRANEAN CHICKPEA AND BULGUR SALAD

Preparation Time: 15 minutes Servings: 4

Nutrition per Serving: Calories: 230, Carbs: 40g, Protein: 10g, Fat: 5g

Ingredients:

- 1 cup bulgur, cooked
- 1 can chickpeas (low sodium), drained
- 1 cucumber, diced
- 1 cup cherry tomatoes, halved

3. Pressure cook on high for 15 minutes.

- 2 tbsp. feta cheese, crumbled
- 1/4 cup Kalamata olives, sliced
- 2 tbsp. olive oil
- 1 tsp dried oregano
- Salt and pepper to taste

Instructions:

1. In a large bowl, combine bulgur, chickpeas, cucumber, cherry tomatoes, olives, and feta.
2. In a small bowl, whisk together olive oil, dried oregano, salt, and pepper. Pour over the salad.

Preparation Time: 20 minutes Servings: 4

Nutrition per Serving: Calories: 250, Carbs: 45g, Protein: 10g, Fat: 5g

Ingredients:

- 2 sweet potatoes, baked
- 1 cup quinoa, cooked
- 1 can black beans (low sodium), drained
- 1 cup corn kernels (fresh or frozen)
- 1 avocado, sliced
- 1/4 cup cilantro, chopped
- 1 lime, juiced
- Salt and pepper to taste

Instructions:

1. Cut baked sweet potatoes in half.
2. In a bowl, mix quinoa, black beans, corn, cilantro, lime juice, salt, and pepper.
3. Stuff sweet potatoes with the quinoa mixture and top with avocado slices.

SNACKS AND APPETIZERS:

QUINOA AND BLACK BEAN STUFFED PEPPERS

Preparation Time: 20 minutes Servings: 8

Nutrition per Serving: Calories: 150, Carbs: 20g, Protein: 5g, Fat: 6g

Ingredients:

- 4 bell peppers, halved and seeded
- 1 cup quinoa, cooked
- 1 can black beans (low sodium), drained
- 1 cup corn kernels
- 1 cup cherry tomatoes, diced
- 1/2 cup red onion, finely chopped
- 1/4 cup cilantro, chopped
- Juice of 1 lime
- Salt and pepper to taste

Instructions:

1. In a bowl, mix cooked quinoa, black beans, corn, tomatoes, red onion, cilantro, lime juice, salt, and pepper.
2. Stuff the pepper halves with the mixture.
3. Place in the Instant Pot with 1 cup of water.
4. Pressure cook for 5 minutes.

SPINACH AND ARTICHOKE DIP

Preparation Time: 15 minutes Servings: 10

Nutrition per Serving: Calories: 120, Carbs: 5g, Protein: 4g, Fat: 8g

Ingredients:

- 2 cups frozen chopped spinach, thawed and drained
- 1 can artichoke hearts, drained and chopped
- 1 cup plain Greek yogurt
- 1 cup cream cheese (light), softened
- 1 cup grated Parmesan cheese
- 1 cup mozzarella cheese, shredded
- 2 cloves garlic, minced
- Salt and pepper to taste

Instructions:

1. In the Instant Pot, combine spinach, artichoke hearts, Greek yogurt, cream cheese, Parmesan, mozzarella, garlic, salt, and pepper.
2. Mix well and pressure cook on high for 5 minutes.

EGG MUFFINS WITH TURKEY AND VEGGIES

Preparation Time: 15 minutes Servings: 6

Nutrition per Serving: Calories: 120, Carbs: 3g, Protein: 15g, Fat: 5g

Ingredients:

- 6 eggs, beaten
- 1/2 lb ground turkey, cooked
- 1 cup bell peppers, diced
- 1 cup spinach, chopped
- 1/2 cup cherry tomatoes, halved
- 1/4 cup feta cheese, crumbled
- 1 tsp olive oil
- Salt and pepper to taste

Instructions:

1. In a bowl, mix beaten eggs, cooked turkey, bell peppers, spinach, tomatoes, feta cheese, salt, and pepper.
2. Grease muffin tin with olive oil and pour the mixture into each cup.
3. Pressure cook on high for 8 minutes.

CAPRESE SALAD SKEWERS

Preparation Time: 10 minutes Servings: 6

Nutrition per Serving: Calories: 80, Carbs: 4g, Protein: 3g, Fat: 6g

Ingredients:

- 1 pint cherry tomatoes
- 1 package fresh mozzarella balls
- Fresh basil leaves
- Balsamic glaze for drizzling
- Salt and pepper to taste

- 1/2 tsp paprika

Instructions:

1. Thread cherry tomatoes, mozzarella balls, and basil leaves onto skewers.
2. Arrange skewers in the Instant Pot.
3. Pressure cook on high for 1 minute.
4. Drizzle with balsamic glaze before serving.

CAULIFLOWER BUFFALO BITES

Preparation Time: 15 minutes Servings: 4

Nutrition per Serving: Calories: 100, Carbs: 8g, Protein: 4g, Fat: 6g

Ingredients:

- 1 small head cauliflower, cut into florets
- 1/2 cup almond flour
- 1/2 cup unsweetened almond milk
- 1 tsp garlic powder
- 1 tsp onion powder
- 1/2 cup buffalo sauce (sugar free)

Instructions:

1. In a bowl, mix almond flour, almond milk, garlic powder, and onion powder.
2. Dip cauliflower florets into the batter and place them on a trivet in the Instant Pot.
3. Pressure cook on high for 3 minutes.
4. Toss with buffalo sauce before serving.

ZUCCHINI AND PARMESAN BITES

Preparation Time: 15 minutes Servings: 4

Nutrition per Serving: Calories: 90, Carbs: 5g, Protein: 5g, Fat: 6g

Ingredients:

- 2 zucchinis, sliced into rounds
- 1/2 cup grated Parmesan cheese
- 1/4 cup almond flour
- 1 tsp Italian seasoning
- Olive oil for brushing

Instructions:

1. In a bowl, mix Parmesan cheese, almond flour, and Italian seasoning.
2. Dip zucchini slices into the mixture and place them on a trivet in the Instant Pot.
3. Brush with olive oil.
4. Pressure cook on high for 5 minutes.

SWEET POTATO AND CHICKPEA PATTIES

Preparation Time: 20 minutes Servings: 6

Nutrition per Serving: Calories: 150, Carbs: 20g, Protein: 5g, Fat: 6g

Ingredients:

- 2 medium sweet potatoes, peeled and grated
- 1 can chickpeas (low sodium), drained
- 1/2 cup breadcrumbs (whole wheat)
- 1/4 cup parsley, chopped
- 1 tsp cumin
- Olive oil for greasing

Instructions:

1. In a food processor, blend sweet potatoes, chickpeas, breadcrumbs, parsley, cumin, and paprika until well combined.
2. Shape the mixture into patties and place them on a greased trivet in the Instant Pot.
3. Pressure cook on high for 8 minutes.

MANGO SALSA

Preparation Time: 10 minutes Servings: 8

Nutrition per Serving: Calories: 40, Carbs: 10g, Protein: 1g, Fat: 0g

Ingredients:

- 2 mangoes, diced
- 1 red onion, finely chopped
- 1 red bell pepper, diced
- 1 jalapeño, seeded and minced
- 1/4 cup fresh cilantro, chopped
- Juice of 2 limes
- Salt and pepper to taste

Instructions:

1. In a bowl, combine mangoes, red onion, red bell pepper, jalapeño, cilantro, lime juice, salt, and pepper.
2. Place the bowl on a trivet in the Instant Pot.
3. Pressure cook on high for 2 minutes.

BRUSSELS SPROUTS CHIPS

Preparation Time: 15 minutes Servings: 4

Nutrition per Serving: Calories: 60, Carbs: 8g, Protein: 3g, Fat: 3g

Ingredients:

- 1 lb. Brussels sprouts, trimmed and halved
- 1 tbsp. olive oil
- 1/2 tsp garlic powder
- 1/2 tsp onion powder
- Salt and pepper to taste

Instructions:

1. Toss Brussels sprouts with olive oil, garlic powder, onion powder, salt, and pepper.
2. Arrange in a single layer on a trivet in the Instant Pot.
3. Pressure cook on high for 3 minutes.

AVOCADO AND BLACK BEAN SALSA

Preparation Time: 10 minutes Servings: 6

Nutrition per Serving: Calories: 90, Carbs: 10g, Protein: 2g, Fat: 6g

Ingredients:

- 2 avocados, diced
- 1 can black beans (low sodium), drained
- 1 cup corn kernels
- 1/2 red onion, finely chopped
- 1/4 cup fresh cilantro, chopped
- Juice of 1 lime
- Salt and pepper to taste

Instructions:

1. In a bowl, combine avocados, black beans, corn, red onion, cilantro, lime juice, salt, and pepper.
2. Place the bowl on a trivet in the Instant Pot.
3. Pressure cook on high for 2 minutes.

CUCUMBER AND TZATZIKI BITES

Preparation Time: 15 minutes Servings: 4

Nutrition per Serving: Calories: 70, Carbs: 5g, Protein: 3g, Fat: 4g

Ingredients:

- 2 cucumbers, sliced
- 1 cup Greek yogurt
- 1/2 cup cucumber, finely chopped
- 2 tbsp fresh dill, chopped
- 1 clove garlic, minced
- Salt and pepper to taste

Instructions:

1. In a bowl, mix Greek yogurt, chopped cucumber, dill, garlic, salt, and pepper to make tzatziki sauce.
2. Top cucumber slices with tzatziki sauce.
3. Place them on a trivet in the Instant Pot.
4. Pressure cook on high for 2 minutes.

STUFFED MUSHROOMS WITH FETA AND SPINACH

Preparation Time: 15 minutes Servings: 6

Nutrition per Serving: Calories: 70,Carbs: 5g, Protein: 4g, Fat: 4g

Ingredients:

- 12 large mushrooms, cleaned and stems removed
- 1 cup spinach, chopped
- 1/2 cup feta cheese, crumbled
- 1/4 cup red bell pepper, finely chopped
- 2 cloves garlic, minced
- 1 tbsp olive oil
- Salt and pepper to taste

Instructions:

1. In a pan, sauté spinach, feta, red bell pepper, garlic, salt, and pepper in olive oil until wilted.
2. Stuff mushrooms with the mixture.
3. Place on a trivet in the Instant Pot.
4. Pressure cook for 5 minutes.

CHICKEN LETTUCE WRAPS

Preparation Time: 20 minutes Servings: 4

Nutrition per Serving: Calories: 160, Carbs: 10g, Protein: 20g, Fat: 5g

Ingredients:

- 1 lb. ground chicken
- 1 cup water chestnuts, chopped
- 1/2 cup carrots, julienned
- 2 cloves garlic, minced
- 2 tbsp. low sodium soy sauce
- 1 tbsp. hoisin sauce
- 1 tsp ginger, grated
- 1/4 cup green onions, sliced
- Butter lettuce leaves for wrapping

Instructions:

1. In the Instant Pot, sauté ground chicken until cooked.
2. Add water chestnuts, carrots, garlic, soy sauce, hoisin sauce, and ginger. Cook for an additional 5 minutes.
3. Spoon the mixture into lettuce leaves.

CRISPY CHICKPEAS

Preparation Time: 10 minutes Servings: 4

Nutrition per Serving: Calories: 80, Carbs: 12g, Protein: 4g, Fat: 2g

Ingredients:

- 2 cans chickpeas (low sodium), drained and rinsed
- 1 tbsp. olive oil
- 1 tsp smoked paprika
- 1/2 tsp cumin
- Salt and pepper to taste

Instructions:

1. Toss chickpeas with olive oil, smoked paprika, cumin, salt, and pepper.
2. Place in a single layer on a trivet in the Instant Pot.
3. Pressure cook on high for 5 minutes.

MEDITERRANEAN HUMMUS

Preparation Time: 10 minutes Servings: 8

Nutrition per Serving: Calories: 80, Carbs: 8g, Protein: 3g, Fat: 4g

Ingredients:

- 2 cans chickpeas (low sodium), drained
- 1/4 cup tahini
- 2 cloves garlic, minced
- Juice of 1 lemon
- 2 tbsp. olive oil
- 1 tsp cumin
- Salt and pepper to taste
- Paprika for garnish

Instructions:

1. In a food processor, blend chickpeas, tahini, garlic, lemon juice, olive oil, cumin, salt, and pepper until smooth.
2. Transfer to a serving bowl, drizzle with extra olive oil, and sprinkle with paprika.

BUFFALO CAULIFLOWER BITES

Preparation Time: 15 minutes Servings: 4

Nutrition per Serving: Calories: 70, Carbs: 10g, Protein: 3g, Fat: 3g

Ingredients:

- 1 head cauliflower, cut into florets
- 1/2 cup almond flour
- 1/2 cup unsweetened almond milk
- 1/2 cup buffalo sauce (sugar free)
- 1 tbsp. olive oil
- Ranch dressing for dipping

Instructions:

1. In a bowl, mix almond flour and almond milk.
2. Dip cauliflower florets into the batter and place them on a trivet in the Instant Pot.
3. Pressure cook on high for 3 minutes.
4. Toss with buffalo sauce before serving and serve with ranch dressing.

TOMATO BASIL BRUSCHETTA

Preparation Time: 10 minutes Servings: 6

Nutrition per Serving: Calories: 60, Carbs: 8g, Protein: 2g, Fat: 2g

Ingredients:

- 4 tomatoes, diced
- 1/4 cup fresh basil, chopped
- 2 cloves garlic, minced
- 1 tbsp balsamic vinegar
- 2 tbsp olive oil
- Salt and pepper to taste
- Baguette slices for serving

Instructions:

- In a bowl, combine tomatoes, basil, garlic, balsamic vinegar, olive oil, salt, and pepper.
- Toast baguette slices in the Instant Pot using the sauté function.
- Serve the bruschetta on top of the toasted baguette slices.
-

CILANTRO LIME CAULIFLOWER RICE

Preparation Time: 15 minutes Servings: 6

Nutrition per Serving: Calories: 60, Carbs: 5g, Protein: 2g, Fat: 4g

Ingredients:

- 1 head cauliflower, riced
- 1/4 cup fresh cilantro, chopped
- Juice of 2 limes
- 1 tbsp. olive oil
- Salt and pepper to taste

Instructions:

1. In the Instant Pot, sauté riced cauliflower in olive oil until slightly golden.
2. Stir in chopped cilantro, lime juice, salt, and pepper.
3. Pressure cook on high for 2 minutes.

GREEK SALAD

Preparation Time: 10 minutes Servings: 4

Nutrition per Serving: Calories: 100, Carbs: 10g, Protein: 3g, Fat: 6g

Ingredients:

- 2 cucumbers, diced
- 2 tomatoes, diced
- 1/2 cup Kalamata olives, sliced
- 1/2 cup feta cheese, crumbled
- 1/4 cup red onion, finely chopped
- 1/4 cup fresh parsley, chopped
- 2 tbsp olive oil
- Juice of 1 lemon
- Salt and pepper to taste

Instructions:

1. In a bowl, combine cucumbers, tomatoes, olives, feta, red onion, parsley, olive oil, lemon juice, salt, and pepper.
2. Place the bowl on a trivet in the Instant Pot.
3. Pressure cook on high for 2 minutes.

STUFFED BELL PEPPER DIP

Preparation Time: 15 minutes

Servings: 8

Nutrition per Serving: Calories: 100, Carbs: 8g, Protein: 4g, Fat: 6g

Ingredients:

- 2 bell peppers, diced
- 1 cup ground turkey, cooked
- 1 cup black beans (low sodium), drained
- 1 cup shredded cheddar cheese
- 1/2 cup salsa
- 1 tsp cumin
- 1/2 tsp chili powder
- Salt and pepper to taste

Instructions:

1. In the Instant Pot, combine diced bell peppers, cooked turkey black beans, cheddar cheese, salsa, cumin, chili powder, salt, and pepper.
2. Mix well and pressure cook on high for 5 minutes.

SPICY EDAMAME

Preparation Time: 10 minutes Servings: 4

Nutrition per Serving: Calories: 80, Carbs: 6g, Protein: 6g, Fat: 4g

Ingredients:

- 2 cups edamame (frozen, in shells)
- 1 tbsp. olive oil
- 1 tsp chili powder
- 1/2 tsp garlic powder
- Salt to taste

Instructions:

1. In a bowl, toss edamame with olive oil, chili powder, garlic powder, and salt.
2. Place in a steamer basket in the Instant Pot.
3. Pressure cook on high for 2 minutes.

CUCUMBER AVOCADO ROLLS

Preparation Time: 15 minutes Servings: 4

Nutrition per Serving: Calories: 90, Carbs: 5g, Protein: 2g, Fat: 7g

Ingredients:

- 2 cucumbers, peeled into strips
- 1 avocado, sliced
- 1/2 cup crabmeat (imitation), shredded
- 1/4 cup mayonnaise (light)
- 1 tsp sriracha sauce
- Sesame seeds for garnish

Instructions:

1. Lay cucumber strips flat and spread a thin layer of mayo on each.
2. Place avocado slices and a small amount of shredded crabmeat on each strip.
3. Drizzle with sriracha and roll up the cucumber.
4. Place rolls on a trivet in the Instant Pot.
5. Pressure cook on high for 3 minutes.

SALSA VERDE CHICKEN WINGS

Preparation Time: 15 minutes Servings: 4

Nutrition per Serving: Calories: 200, Carbs: 2g, Protein: 18g, Fat: 12g

Ingredients:

- 2 lbs. chicken wings
- 1 cup salsa verde
- 1/2 cup cilantro, chopped
- 1 tsp cumin
- 1 tsp garlic powder
- Salt and pepper to taste

Instructions:

1. In a bowl, mix chicken wings with salsa verde, cilantro, cumin, garlic powder, salt, and pepper.
2. Place wings on a trivet in the Instant Pot.
3. Pressure cook on high for 10 minutes.

MEXICAN STREET CORN DIP

Preparation Time: 15 minutes Servings: 8

Nutrition per Serving: Calories: 120, Carbs: 15g, Protein: 3g, Fat: 6g

Ingredients:

- 4 cups frozen corn, thawed
- 1 cup cotija cheese, crumbled
- 1/2 cup mayonnaise (light)
- 1/4 cup cilantro, chopped
- 1 tsp chili powder
- 1/2 tsp cayenne pepper
- Juice of 2 limes
- Salt and pepper to taste

Instructions:

1. In the Instant Pot, combine corn, cotija cheese, mayo, cilantro, chili powder, cayenne pepper, lime juice, salt, and pepper.
2. Mix well and pressure cook on high for 5 minutes.

TERIYAKI SALMON BITES

Preparation Time: 15 minutes Servings: 4

Nutrition per Serving: Calories: 180, Carbs: 10g, Protein: 18g, Fat: 8g

Ingredients:

- 1 lb salmon fillet, cut into bite sized pieces
- 1/4 cup low sodium soy sauce
- 2 tbsp. honey
- 1 tbsp. rice vinegar
- 1 tsp sesame oil
- 1 tsp ginger, grated
- 2 cloves garlic, minced
- Green onions for garnish

Instructions:

1. In a bowl, mix salmon, soy sauce, honey, rice vinegar, sesame oil, ginger, and garlic.
2. Place salmon pieces on a trivet in the Instant Pot.
3. Pressure cook on high for 3 minutes.
4. Garnish with chopped green onions before serving.

CONCLUSION

In wrapping up this Diabetes Instant Pot Cookbook, it becomes clear why Instant Pot recipes are a game-changer for individuals managing diabetes. Beyond the convenience and efficiency that the Instant Pot brings to the kitchen, its impact on crafting diabetes-friendly meals is truly transformative.

The allure of Instant Pot recipes lies in their ability to streamline the cooking process without compromising on flavor, nutrition, or variety. The recipes presented in this cookbook showcase how the Instant Pot, with its multi-functionality and time-saving features, can be an invaluable tool for individuals seeking to manage their blood sugar levels effectively.

One of the standout advantages is the speed at which the Instant Pot operates. With busy lifestyles, finding time to prepare wholesome meals can be challenging, but the Instant Pot accelerates the cooking process without sacrificing the nutritional integrity of ingredients. This time efficiency is a crucial factor for those managing diabetes, providing an accessible way to enjoy home-cooked meals even on the busiest days.

The controlled cooking environment of the Instant Pot ensures that flavors are sealed in, allowing for the creation of dishes that are not only healthy but also incredibly delicious. The versatility of the Instant Pot has been showcased across various sections of this cookbook, from breakfast delights to comforting stews and vibrant vegetable dishes. Whether it's hearty soups, flavorful poultry, or seafood sensations, the Instant Pot proves to be a reliable companion in the quest for diverse and enticing meals that align with diabetic dietary guidelines.

Moreover, the Instant Pot's ability to tenderize tough cuts of meat quickly opens up a world of culinary possibilities, allowing for the creation of satisfying and protein-rich dishes. This is particularly significant for individuals managing diabetes, as protein intake plays a crucial role in maintaining stable blood sugar levels.

In essence, this cookbook demonstrates that Instant Pot recipes are not just a practical solution for time-conscious cooks but also a culinary ally for those navigating the intricacies of diabetes management. The joy of savoring well-prepared, wholesome meals should be accessible to everyone, and the Instant Pot proves to be an inclusive tool in achieving this goal.

As you embark on your culinary journey with the Instant Pot, may the recipes in this cookbook bring not only convenience to your kitchen but also a newfound appreciation for the delicious possibilities that await. Here's to nourishing meals, delightful flavors, and the empowering choice to embrace a healthier, more manageable approach to living with diabetes. Happy cooking!

93 Diabetes Instant Pot Cookbook For Beginners

14 DAYS MEAL PLAN

Week 1

Breakfast	Lunch	Snack	Dinner
Chocolate Banana Overnight Oats	Chicken and Vegetable Stir-fry	Pecan Pie Bars:	Turkey Chili
Veggie and Cheese Egg Bites	Lemon Garlic Shrimp:	Mango Coconut Rice Pudding:	Beef and Zucchini Lasagna
Spinach and Mushroom Frittata	Red Lentil and Spinach Soup	Pistachio Orange Biscotti:	Spinach and Mushroom Risotto
Maple Pecan Quinoa	Lamb and Eggplant Curry	Sautéed Lemon Garlic Spinach	Mediterranean Fish Stew:
Avocado and Tomato Egg Cups	Black Bean Soup	Chocolate Covered Strawberry Cups:	Garlic Herb Quinoa
Berry Quinoa Breakfast Bowl	Miso Glazed Cod:	Shrimp and Avocado Salad:	Pinto Bean and Quinoa Chili
Apple Cinnamon Breakfast Rice Pudding	Chicken and Quinoa Casserole	Almond Joy Energy Bites:	Vegetable Lentil Soup

Breakfast	Lunch	Snack	Dinner
Vegetable Frittata	Salsa Verde Chicken Wings	Pecan Pie Bars	Turkey Chili
Cottage Cheese Pancakes	Sweet Potato and Chickpea Stew	Almond Flour Lemon Poppy Seed Muffins	Ratatouille
Greek Yogurt Parfait	Pork and Apple Skillet	Coconut Flour Banana Bread	Mediterranean Chickpea and Bulgur Salad
Berry Oatmeal	Three Bean Quinoa Salad	Chocolate Avocado Mousse:	Lamb and Chickpea Tagine
Pumpkin Spice Oatmeal	Beef and Spinach Stuffed Mushrooms	Spinach and Artichoke Dip	Cilantro Lime Cauliflower Rice
Lemon Poppy Seed Instant Pot Muffins	Quinoa and Black Bean Stuffed Bell Peppers	Hazelnut Chocolate Spread:	Mixed Grain and Vegetable Risotto
Banana Walnut Bread Oatmeal	Barley and Vegetable Soup	Quinoa and Black Bean Stuffed Peppers	Pork and Vegetable Curry